Experimental
Pharmacology

Experimental Pharmacology

DR. K.K. PILLAI, M.Pharm., Ph.D.
Professor and Head
Department of Pharmacology
Faculty of Pharmacy
Jamia Hamdard (Hamdard University)
Hamdard Nagar, New Delhi-110062

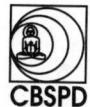

CBS Publishers & Distributors Pvt Ltd

New Delhi • Bengaluru • Chennai • Kochi • Kolkata • Lucknow • Mumbai
Hyderabad • Jharkhand • Nagpur • Patna • Pune • Uttarakhand

Experimental Pharmacology

ISBN: 978-81-239-0649-2

Copyright © Author

First Edition: 1999

Reprint: 2003, 2004, 2005, 2006, 2007, 2008, 2009, 2010, 2012, 2014, 2016, 2018, 2019, 2020, 2023

Published by Satish Kumar Jain and produced by Varun Jain for

CBS Publishers & Distributors Pvt Ltd

4819/XI Prahlad Street, 24 Ansari Road, Daryaganj, New Delhi 110 002, India

Ph: 011-23289259, 23266861, 23266867   Website: www.cbspd.com

Fax: 011-23243014   e-mail: delhi@cbspd.com; cbspubs@airtelmail.in

Corporate Office: 204 FIE, Industrial Area, Patparganj, Delhi 110 092

Ph: 011-4934 4934   Fax: 011-4934 4935   e-mail: publishing@cbspd.com; publicity@cbspd.com

Branches

* **Bengaluru:** Seema House 2975, 17th Cross, KR Road, Banasankari 2nd Stage, Bengaluru 560 070, Karnataka, India
  Ph: +91-80-26771678/79   Fax: +91-80-26771680   e-mail: bangalore@cbspd.com
* **Chennai:** 7, Subbaraya Street, Shenoy Nagar, Chennai 600 030, Tamil Nadu, India
  Ph: +91-44-26680620, 26681266   Fax: +91-44-42032115   e-mail: chennai@cbspd.com
* **Kochi:** 42/1325, 1326, Power House Road, Opp KSEB, Power House, Ernakulam, Kochi 682 018, India
  Ph: +91-484-4059061–65   Fax: +91-484-4059065   e-mail: kochi@cbspd.com
* **Kolkata:** 147, Hind Ceramics Compound, 1st Floor, Nilgunj Road, Belghoria, Kolkata 700 056, West Bengal, India
  Ph: +91-33-25633055–56   e-mail: kolkata@cbspd.com
* **Lucknow:** Basement, Khushnuma Complex, 7-Meerabai Marg (behind Jawahar Bhawan), Lucknow 226 001, India
  Ph: +91-522-4000032   e-mail: tiwari.lucknow@cbspd.com
* **Mumbai:** PWD Shed. Gala no. 25/26, Ramchandra Bhatt Marg, Next to JJ Hospital Gate no. 2, Opp. Union Bank of India, Noorbaug Mumbai 400 009, Maharashtra, India
  Ph: +91-22-66661880/89   e-mail: mumbai@cbspd.com

Representatives

* **Hyderabad** 0-9885175004 * **Jharkhand** 0-9811541605 * **Nagpur** 0-9421945513
* **Patna** 0-9334159340 * **Pune** 0-9623451994 * **Uttarakhand** 0-9716462459

Printed at Neekunj Print Process, Haryana, India

Dedicated to My Parents

Preface

This book is a compilation of specific techniques used in understanding the basic principles of Pharmacology and also the evaluation of potential drugs. I have attempted to bring out a book which stresses a practical and applied approach to biological evaluation techniques. Step-by-step procedures for the identification of unknown compounds for specific pharmacological activity are given in a lucid manner. This gives an opportunity to the investigators to carry out screening procedures of compounds of either known or unknown pharmacological activity. The experiments on bioassay have been written in such a way that a student can perform 25 different experiments on this topic. This book has been compiled from my involvement, for 25 years, in the teaching of Pharmacology practical to Pharmacy undergraduate and post-graduate students in the Department of Pharmacology at the Faculty of Pharmacy, Jamia Hamdard (Hamdard University) at New Delhi. I am sure this book will also be useful to medical and veterinary graduates. I am grateful to Mr. S.K. Jain, Managing Director, CBS Publishers and Distributors for the encouragement and suggestions. Many thanks are extended to Mr. B.R. Sharma and other staff of CBS Publishers for expedicting the production of this book. I would like to thank all my family members who helped me in every possible way. Suggestion from readers is welcomed.

New Delhi   K.K. PILLAI

Abbreviations

Ach	Acetylcholine
AMPA	(DL alpha amino 3-hydroxy-5-methylisoxazole 4 propionate)
GABA	Gamma Amino Butyric Acid
g	gram
mg	Microgram
mg	Milligram
i.m.	Intramuscular
i.v.	Intravenous
MES	Maximal electroshock
M	Molar
p.o.	per oral route
s.c.	Subcutaneous

Contents

CHAPTER 1
Introduction

MEASURING DRUG ACTIVITY

Experimental Pharmacology plays an important role in the identification of new molecules with selective pharmacological activities which may be useful clinically. Drug development is impossible without proper quantitative pharmacological tests. If a drug produces an effect, it changes the properties of some of the cells in an organism. Some effects may be visible but most can only be identified with suitable equipments. Many effects involve physical or chemical changes which can be measured.

PHYSICAL CHANGES

Changes in mechanical properties like change in length, volume, pressure, blood flow and rates of contraction can be measured using multichannel polygraph. Similarly changes in electrical properties like polarization depolarization, hyperpolarization etc. can be measured using specific instruments.

CHEMICAL CHANGES

The levels of biochemicals and enzymes during physiological condition, pathological condition and after treatment with drugs can be measured to find out the influence of new molecules on these parameters.

AIMS OF EXPERIMENTAL PHARMACOLOGY

1. To find out a therapeutic agent suitable for human use.
2. To study the toxicity of a drug.
3. To study the mechanism(s) of action and site(s) of action of drugs.

STUDY OF INSTRUMENTS USED IN EXPERIMENTAL PHARMACOLOGY

In experimental Pharmacology, more sophisticated instruments are introduced in recent years for recording the responses of intact animals and isolated tissues.

Name of the instruments commonly used in the Pharmacology laboratory are given below :

1. Multichannel polygraph is used for recording cardiovascular responses like ECG, blood pressure, heart rate etc. and is also used to record respiration and temperature.

2. Bloodless B.P. apparatus is used to evaluate antihypertensive agents.

3. Research flow meters can be used for both acute and chronic animal studies to monitor :

   (i) Ventricular function

   (ii) Pulmonary function

   (iii) Coronary circulation

   (iv) Renal hypertension

   (v) Nutrient metabolism

   (vi) Microcirculation

   (vii) Lymph flow

   (viii) Fetal blood flow, and

   (ix) Other hemodynamics.

4. Plethysmometer is used to evaluate anti-inflammatory drugs like indomethacin and ketoprofen etc.

5. Analgesiometer, Tail Flick apparatus, Eddys hot plate are widely used to evaluate analgesic activity of a new molecule.

6. Telethermometer (Multichannel Automatic) is used to record temperature of rabbits during pyrogen testing.

7. Airway Narrowing Analyser is useful to evaluate antiasthmatic agents.

8. Histometer is used to evaluate H_1-receptor blocking agents.

9. Electroconvulsometer is used to evaluate anticonvulsant activity.

10. Rota rod is used to evaluate the drugs which affect the motor function.

11. Actophotometer/Photocell counter is used to screen sedative hypnotic agents and also central nervous system stimulants.

12. Cooks pole climbing apparatus is used to evaluate neuroleptics.
13. Elevated Plus-Maze is used to evaluate anti-anxiety agents.
14. Feeding-Monitor is used to evaluate the drugs which affect the feeding behaviour.
15. CMA Microdialysis system is used for metabolic and pharmacokinetic studies. CMA microdialysis system coupled with HPLC or mass spectrometer is used for measuring CNS transmitter like acetylcholine, adrenaline, aspartate, GABA, glutamate, dopamine etc. in different areas of the brain.

CONVENTIONAL EQUIPMENTS USED IN EXPERIMENTAL PHARMACOLOGY

Kymograph

Different models of Kymographs are available. Kymograph is an electrical device consists of gear box with provision for carrying drum. The speed of the drum can be controlled by clutch and gear. While setting up the assembly for any experiment care has to be taken to ensure that the Kymograph cylinder is strictly perpendicular to the working bench and that the lever moves in the same vertical lane. If the Kymograph is not kept perpendicular to the working bench, the lever will either leave the paper at some point in its excursion or it will press more heavily at some points on the paper and increased friction will retard the movements.

Organ baths

Organ bath is an assembly for recording either contraction or relaxation of isolated tissues. The design of organ bath varies from laboratory to laboratory. It may be a single unit as designed by Rudolph Magnus or a double unit as designed by Sir Gaddum. The various parts of organ bath are as follows :

(i) A rectangular outer bath made up of perspex. A thermostate and heating element are also fixed with the outer bath. An electrically operated stirrer is also fixed in the outer organ bath of the newly designed single unit organ bath.

(ii) An inner organ bath made up of glass has capacity around 50 ml. The inner organ bath has inlet and outlet for the physiological solution. The inlet side tube is connected to a glass coil. The other end of the coil is connected to the Mariotte bottle through polythene tube.

(iii) Two small perpendicular rods attached both at left side and right side of the outer organ bath are used for fixing the frontal writing lever and aeration tube respectively.

(iv) The hook of the aeration tube also acts as a tissue holder.

Precaution

The outer organ bath should be filled with water before connecting the organ bath to the electrical points.

Maintenance of organ bath

1. The inner organ bath should always be washed with distilled water after use to prevent the growth of fungus and other microorganisms.

2. The inner organ both should be periodically cleaned with hydrochloric acid or chromic acid.

Mariotte bottle
(Mariotte—A French Physiologist)

Mariotte bottle is used to keep the physiological solutions used in the experiment.

Maintenance of Mariotte bottle

The Mariotte-bottle should be periodically cleaned with hydrochloric acid or chromic acid.

Recording devices

Levers are used for recording either contraction or relaxation of tissues. Types of levers used in the experimental pharmacology are :

(a) Class I type mechanical lever

In class I lever the fulcrum or pivot lies between the writing point and the point of attachment of the tissue e.g. Frontal writing lever.

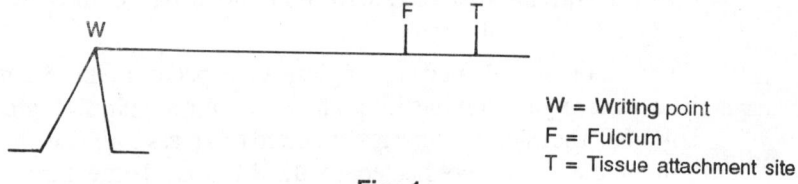

W = Writing point
F = Fulcrum
T = Tissue attachment site

Fig. 1.

Frontal writing lever is an isotonic lever. It allows the tissue to contract freely against a constant tension. Therefore, the recording is called isotonic recording. The writing point of the frontal writing lever rotates freely about its axle. Hence, recordings are done on the smoked paper of the drum without much friction.

(b) Class II type lever

In class II lever the fulcrum lies at one end beyond the point of attachment of the tissue e.g. Starling's heart lever.

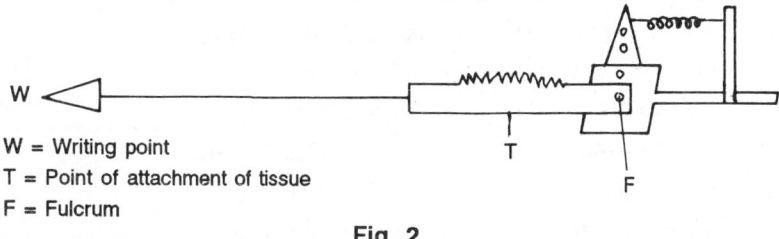

W = Writing point
T = Point of attachment of tissue
F = Fulcrum

Fig. 2.

Adjustment for magnification

In order to magnify the actual contraction response of the tissue, the lever should be adjusted properly. The distance between the Fulcrum (F) and the writing point should be greater than the distance between the fulcrum and the point of attachment of the tissue.

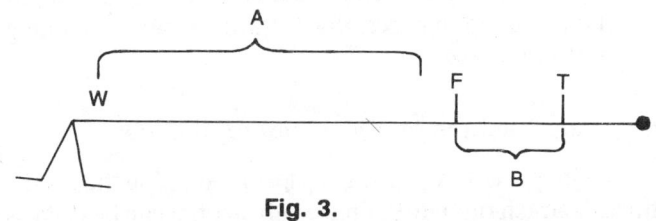

Fig. 3.

$$\text{Magnification value} = \frac{\text{Distance between fulcrum and writing point (A)}}{\text{Distance between fulcrum and the point of attachment to the tissue (B)}}$$

The tissues showing less contractility (e.g. Frog rectus abdominis muscle) needs five times to ten times magnification. Rat uterus muscle requires 2-4 times magnification. Guinea pig ileum needs 5-7 times magnification.

Adjustment of load or tension on frontal writing lever

Balance the frontal writing lever by placing sufficient plasticine on the shorter arm near the end of the lever. This is done because the fulcrum is usually away from the mid point. Then, place the prescribed weight on the balanced lever exactly at the site of attachment to the tissue. Fix small quantity of plasticine (equal to the prescribed weight) on the longer arm of the lever so that distance between the fulcrum and the point of attachment of tension (load) is equal to the distance between the fulcrum and the point of attachment to the tissue. After mounting the tissue in the organ bath remove the prescribed weight from the point of attachment to the tissue and attach the thread of the tissue.

The load prescribed for various tissues are as follows :

Frog rectus abdominis muscle	1 gram
Guinea pig ileum	500 milligram
Rat intestine	500 milligram
Rat uterus	500 milligram
Rabbit intestine	500 milligram to 1 gram
Rat fundus	1 gram

Smoking of drums

The Kymograph graph paper has a glossy surface and a non-glossy surface. The paper should be wrapped round the drum (glossy surface out) and fixed with gum. Using a kerosene burner smoke the glossy surface of the kymograh paper. Rotate the drum while smoking in order to get a uniform smoke.

Fixing of the tracings on the kymograph paper

Fix the tracings on the kymograph paper by dipping the paper in fixing solutions. Varnish diluted 10 times with alcohol can be used as a fixing solution or a saturated solution of colophony in ethylalcohol or methylalcohol can be used as a fixing solution.

Physiological salt solutions for isolated tissues

All physiological salt solutions are prepared in distilled water using Analar Grade Chemicals. Physiological solutions are prepared fresh and used within 24 hours. Storage is not recommended because of the problems of microbial growth. While preparing the physiological salt solution, calcium chloride should be added last in the form of solution in order to prevent the precipitation of bicarbonate. Because isolated tissue will not survive for long periods in cloudy physiological salt solution. Cloudy physiological solution also gives erratic response with drugs. The composition of physiological salt solution which are commonly used in the laboratory are given below.

Composition of physiological salt solution (salts in g/litre)

Name of the ingredients	Name of the physiological salt solutions				
	Frog ringer	Tyrode	De Jalon	Ringer-Locke	Krebs
NaCl	6.5	8	9	9	6.9
NaHCO$_3$	0.2	1	0.5	0.2	2.1
D-glucose	2	1	0.5	1	2
KH$_2$PO$_4$	—	—	—	—	0.16
NaH$_2$PO$_4$	0.01	0.05	—	—	—
KCl	0.14	0.2	0.42	0.42	0.36
MgSO$_4$.7H$_2$O	—	—	—	—	0.29
MgCl$_2$	—	0.1	—	—	—
CaCl$_2$	0.12	0.2	0.06	0.24	0.28
Distilled water to make up volume upto	1000 ml	1000 ml	1000 ml	1000 ml	1000 ml

Role of each chemical in the physiological salt solution

Sodium chloride is required to maintain isotonicity. Sodium chloride and potassium chloride maintain the membrane potential. Sodium bicarbonate maintains the alkaline pH. Potassium dihydrogen phosphate or sodium dihydrogen phosphate act as buffer. Magnesium chloride or Magnesium sulphate play a role in the relaxation of smooth muscle. Calcium ions are required for contraction process. Glucose provides energy for the cell.

Handling of laboratory animals

Treat the animals humanely. Do not cause unnecessary discomfort to the animals.

Housing and feeding of experimental animals

Experimental animals should be kept in well maintained animal house. The animal house should have all electrical appliances (Air conditioner, Air cooler, Exhaust fan, Room heaters etc.) so that the temperature of the animal house is maintained between 20-25°C during all seasons of the year.

Animals should be kept on standard pelletized food and given filtered drinking water adlibitum.

Characteristics of laboratory animals

Characteristic	Name of the animals			
	Guinea pig	Mouse	Rabbit	Rat
Daily food intake	50 g	5 g	150-300 g	10-20 g
Puberty	60-70 days	35 days	4 months	40-60 days
Breeding time	Throughout year	Throughout year	May to September	Throughout year
Pregnancy period	63 days	19-20 days	28-36 days	21-23 days
Life span	7-8 years	2-3 years	8 years	2-3 years
Age suitable for experimentation	3 months	20 days	6 months	45 days
Body temperature	37.8-39.5°C	37.9-39.2°C	38.5-39.5°C	37.7-38.8°C
Heart rate (beats/ minute)	260-400	330-780	130-300	300-500
Blood pressure	77/47 S/D	147/106 S/D	110/80 S/D	130/95 S/D
Respiratory rate per minute	100-150	136-216	50-60	100-150
Hemoglobin g%	8-15	10-19	8-15	12-17
RBC (million/cumm)	5-6	4.9-12.5	4.5-7	7.2-9.6
WBC (thousand/ cumm)	4-11	4-12	6-13	6-12
Blood volume % body weight	6	7.5	5	7.5
Body surface area	$K.\sqrt[3]{g^2}$	$K.\sqrt[3]{g^2}$	$K.\sqrt[3]{g^2}$	$K.\sqrt[3]{g^2}$
	K = 8.8 g = body weight in gram	K = 11.4 g = body weight in gram	K = 12.88 g = body weight in gram	K = 9.13 g = body weight in gram

Fasting of experimental animals

Overnight fasting of experimental animals before performing the experiments reduces further biological variation.

Cleanliness of animal house

There should be separate facility for cleaning the animal cages and the animal room should be kept clean always. Animal feed should be stored properly.

Disposal of sacrificed animals

An incinerator can be used to dispose the sacrificed animals and other waste from the animal house.

Code for identifying the animals

It is necessary to identify individual animal of a group or those housed in one cage. To identify individual animals the markings are done with picric acid solution (10% aqueous solution of picric acid).

Administration of drugs to laboratory animals

Syringes and needles

Syringes and needles must be sterile for use in rabbits, guinea pigs and dogs. They need not be sterile but should be extremely clean for use in rats and mice.

Maximum volume of drug solution to be given to animals

Volume in ml

	Intravenous	*Intramuscular*	*Intraperitoneal*	*Subcutaneous*	*Oral*
Mouse	0.5	0.05	1	0.5-1	1
Rat	1	0.1	2-5	2-5	5
Guinea pig	1	0.25	2-5	5	10
Rabbit	5-10	C.5	10-20	5-10	20
Dog	10-20	5	20-50	10	100

Techniques of drug administration in animals

Oral administration

Special feeding needle with ball-shaped end is required to administer solutions or suspension to rats and mice. Special mouth blocks are required to feed guinea pigs or rabbits.

Intravenous

Rabbit : Marginal ear vein is preferred.

Rat, mice : Tail vein is preferred.

Dog : Cephalic vein is preferred.

Intraperitoneal : The drug is administered into the peritoneal region.

Animals used in experimental pharmacology

Albino rat (Rattus norvegicus)

Adult body weight is between 150-200 g. Two strains of albino rats are commonly used in experimental pharmacology.

(i) Wistar strain

(ii) Sprague Dawley.

Wistar strain

Its body length is longer than tail length. It has wide head. It is not susceptible to infection.

Sprague dawley

Its body length is almost equal to tail length. It has long and narrower head. It is susceptible to infection.

Rats do not have gall bladder, tonsil and vomiting centre.

Albino rats are widely used for testing analgesics, antianxiety agents, anticonvulsants, antipyretics, antifertility agents, antidepressants, antihepatotoxic agents, antihypertensive agents, antiulcer drugs and neuroleptics. They are also used for the bioassay of ACTH (Adreno Cortico Tropic Hormone). They are also used for testing the toxicity of a new molecule. The following isolated tissues of rats are also used in experimental pharmacology.

Anococcygeus muscle

Used for the identification of nor adrenaline, 5-hydroxytryptamine and acetylcholine.

Rat colon (descending) : For the identification of nor-adrenaline, substance P, Angiotensin and Prostaglandin $F_2\alpha$.

Rat duodenum : For testing brady-kinin and substance P.

Rat fundus : For the estimation of 5-hydroxytryptamine.

Rat phrenic nerve diaphragm : For the bioassay of d-tubocurarine and other neuromuscular blocking agents.

Rat uterus : For the bioassay of oxytocin and adrenaline.

Albinomouse (Musmusculus)

Adult body weight is 20-25 g. Different strains are available for experimental use. They are widely used for the evaluation of analgesic agents, anticonvulsants, antidepressants, antihepatotoxic agents, neuroleptics, sedative hypnotic agents and antiparkinsonian agents. Mice are widely used for blind screening of new molecules since the body weight of the mouse is very less. Mice are preferred for acute toxicity tests. To find out the carcinogenic and teratogenic nature of a new chemical or drug mice are used. Mice are used to carry out the bioassay of insulin and also to find out the toxicity of biological products like toxins, vaccines etc.

Cat (Feliscatus)

Cat is used to evaluate the drugs acting on the cardiovascular system. Neuromuscular blocking agents are also evaluated using cat. Spinal cat is used for the bioassay of adrenaline.

Albino rabbit (oryctolagus cuniculus)

Adult body weight is between 1.5 to 2 kg. Rabbits are used for the evaluation of antidiabetic agents, local anaesthetics (surface anaesthetic agents), teratogenic agents and drugs acting on reproductive system. They are also used for testing skin irritants. Rabbits are used for the bioassay of insulin and d-tubocurarine. Some species have atropine esterase enzyme in their blood and liver which destroys atropine therefore, they tolerate large doses of atropine. The following isolated tissues of rabbits are used in experimental pharmacology.

Aortic strips : For the identification of alpha receptor agonists.

Heart : For the identification of beta-receptor agonists, beta-receptor blockers, muscarinic receptor agonists and antagonists.

Jejunum or ileum : For the identification of spasmogenic and spasmolytic agents.

Perfused ear artery : For testing nanogram quantity of nor-adrenaline.

Guinea pig (cavia porcellus)

Adult body weight is between 500-800 g. Guinea pigs are widely used for the evaluation of antiasthmatic agents, antihistaminics, antitubercular drugs, local anaesthetics and skin irritants. They are used for the study of Type-I hypersensitivity reactions, ascorbic acid metabolism and also for the bioassay of digitalis preparations.

The following isolated tissues of guinea pig are used in experimental pharmacology.

Guinea pig ileum : For the bioassay of histamine, identification of H_1-receptor agonists and antagonists, muscarinic receptor agonists and antagonists and 5-hydroxytryptamine activity.

Guinea pig tracheal chain : For the evaluation of beta-receptor agonists.

Hamster

Two species are usually used in experimental pharmacology :

1. Syrian or Golden hamster. Adult body weight 80-90 g.
2. Chinese hamster. Adult body weight 35-40 g.

They are used for the evaluation of antidiabetic agents, cytotoxic agents and immunomodulating drugs. They are also used in nutrition studies. Isolated stomach strips are used for the bioassay of prostaglandin E and F.

Dog (canisfamiliaris)

Dogs are used for the evaluation of antidiabetic agents, antiulcer drugs and drugs acting on the cardiovascular system.

Monkey (Macaca mulatta)

Monkeys are used for the evaluation of psychopharmacological agents, immunomodulating agents and drugs affecting reproductive function.

Frog (Ranatigrina)

Frogs are used for the evaluation of local anaesthetics. The following isolated tissues of frog are used in experimental pharmacology.

Isolated frog heart : For the identification of beta-receptor agonists and antagonists, muscarinic receptor agonists and antagonists, cardiac glycosides, potassium ions, calcium ions and calcium channel blockers.

Rectus abdominis muscle : For the identification of nicotinic receptor agonists and antagonists and also anticholine esterase agents.

CHAPTER 2
Routes of Administration of Drugs

EXPERIMENT 1

Influence of routes of administration on drug response

AIM

To find out the onset of action and duration of action of pentobarbitone sodium given by oral route, intraperitoneal route and intravenous route.

PRINCIPLE

Drugs can be applied upon or given into the body through various routes or channels. Route of administration is one of the factors which affect the drug response. When a drug is given through oral route, the onset of pharmacological action is slow. However, the same drug when given by parenteral route produces a rapid onset of action and the intensity of action will also vary.

REQUIREMENTS

Animal :   Mice.

Drug solution :   Pentobarbitone sodium 4.5 mg/mL.

Needle :   Oral feeding needle. 26 No. needle.

Plastic cages - 3.

PROCEDURE

1. Select 15 albino mice having body weight between 25-30 g.
2. Fast the mice for 12 hours before the experiment.
3. Divide the mice into three groups of five animals.
4. Weigh the mouse in each group, do the marking and keep them in plastic cages.

5. Administer the drug solutions as given below :

Group I : Pentobarbitone sodium 45 mg/kg p.o.

Group II : Pentobarbitone sodium 45 mg/kg i.p.

Group III : Pentobarbitone sodium 45 mg/kg i.v.

6. Record the observations as shown below.

Group I : Pentobarbitone sodium 45 mg/kg p.o.

S.	Marking	Body weight	Dose	Time of injection	Observations Loss of LRR	Recovery from LRR	Duration of LRR
1.							
2.							
3.							
4.							
5.							

LRR = loss of righting reflex.

7. Make similar tables for Group II and Group III.

OBSERVATIONS AND CONCLUSION

1. The group I which received pentobarbitone sodium orally did not sleep immediately. Sedation was observed in all animals.

2. When pentobarbitone sodium was given by intraperitoneal route, loss of righting reflex was observed in all mice within five minutes period.

3. When pentobarbitone sodium was given by intravenous route, loss of righting reflex was observed in all animals within 3 minutes period.

4. The above observations indicate that route of administration is one of the factors which influence the drug response.

CHAPTER 3

Experiments on Cardiovascular System

EXPERIMENT 2

Effect of adrenaline, acetylcholine, potassium and calcium on frog heart.

AIM

To study the effects of adrenaline, acetylcholine, potassium chloride and calcium chloride on isolated frog's heart.

PRINCIPLE

Heart is supplied by autonomic nervous system. Adrenaline acts as an agonist. It acts on beta-receptors and increases heart rate and amplitude. Acetylcholine acts on muscarinic receptors as an agonist and decreases the heart rate and amplitude. Excess concentration of potassium chloride stops the heart beat during diastolic phase. Calcium ion excess concentration stops the heart beat during systolic phase. Potassium and calcium ion act on cardiac muscle through non-receptor mechanism of action.

EQUIPMENTS AND OTHER ITEMS REQUIRED

INCO kymograph, starling heart lever, L-stand T-rod, X-blocks, Syme's cannula, screw clip Mariotte bottle, rubber tubes, tuberculine syringe 26 No. needle, surgical instrument box.

Animal required : Frog.

Physiological solutions required : Frog Ringer solution.

Drug solutions required

1. Adrenaline hydrochloride 10 microgram/mL in distilled water.
2. Acetylcholine hydrochloride 10 microgram/mL in distilled water.
3. Potassium chloride 4 per cent in distilled water.
4. Calcium chloride 4 per cent in distilled water.

PROCEDURE

1. Set up the assembly for the above mentioned experiment.

2. Pith a frog by passing a needle through the occipito-atlantic junction between the brain and spinal cord. The stretching out of limbs indicate that the pithing is proper.

3. Place the frog in a tray with the ventral side facing up.

4. Make an incision of the skin longitudinally and then expose the rectus muscle.

5. Make incision around the rectus muscle without damaging the anterior abdominal vein.

6. Expose the heart after cutting the sternum.

7. Remove the pericardial membrane.

8. Tie one side of the aorta.

9. Put a knot around the inferior vena cava then make a small cut for cannulation.

10. After cannulation with Syme's cannula, cut the other side of the aorta and isolate the heart from the body and perfuse with frog Ringer solution. Adjust the flow of the frog Ringer solution through the horizontal arm of the Syme's cannula.

11. Place a heart-clip on the apex of the heart and connect it to a starling heart lever.

12. Record the normal heart beat on a smoked drum.

13. Inject 0.05-0.1 ml of adrenaline solution into the Syme's cannula. Immediately switch on the kymograph and record the effect of adrenaline for 2 minutes period. After 2 minutes switch off the kymograph till the heart beat and amplitude comes to normal. Observe the onset and duration of action of adrenaline.

14. Inject 0.05-0.1 ml of acetylcholine solution into the Syme's cannula. Immediately switch on the kymograph and record the effect of acetylcholine for 2 minutes. After 2 minutes switch off the kymograph till the heart beat and amplitude comes to normal. Observe the onset and duration of action of acetylcholine.

15. Inject 0.1 ml of potassium chloride solution into the Syme's cannula. Immediately switch on the kymograph and record the effect of potassium chloride for 2 minutes period. After 2 minutes switch off the kymograph till the heart beat and amplitude comes to normal. Observe the onset and duration of action of potassium chloride.

16. Inject 0.1 to 0.4 ml of calcium chloride solution into the Syme's cannula. Immediately switch on the kymograph and record the

effect of calcium chloride for 3 minutes period. After 3 minutes switch off the kymograph till the heart beat and amplitude comes to normal. Observe the onset and duration of action of calcium chloride.

OBSERVATION AND CONCLUSION

1. Adrenaline increases the heart rate and amplitude. Heart contains beta-receptors. Adrenaline stimulates beta-receptors and increases the heart rate and amplitude. Based upon this experimental observation, adrenaline 1 in 10,000 solution is recommended in a dose of 10 ml by intravenous infusion for cardiac arrest. Drugs which block beta-receptors (propranolol, atendol etc) are clinically used in hypertension and tachycardia.

2. Acetylcholine decreases the heart rate and amplitude. This effect is similar to the effect produced by vagus nerve stimulation. This effect is mediated through muscarinic receptors. Hence, muscarinic blockers (Atropine, belladonna extract) are used to reduce vagal tone and mucarinic actions.

3. Potassium excess concentration decreases the heart rate and amplitude.

4. Calcium concentration in excess stop the heart beat during systolic phase, an effect similar to digoxin poisoning. Therefore, EDTA (Ethylene diamine tetra-aceticacid) is used in digitalis poisoning. Calcium channel blockers like verapamil, diltiazem, amlodipine etc. are used as antihypertensive agents.

Things to remember

The following drugs are available for disorders of cardiovascular system.

Beta-receptor blocking agents (beta 1-selective)

1. **Atenolol (Tenormin, Aloten, Angitol, Atecard, Atelol, Aten, Atenova, Betacard, Betanol) :**

   Oral : 25, 50, 75, 100 mg tablets.

   Dose : For hypertension, 50 mg once in a day maximum 100 mg/day.

   For acute myocardial infarction : 50-100 mg once in a day.

   Atenolol is also used in thyrotoxicosis, left ventricular hypertrophy and pregnancy induced hypertension.

2. **Metoprolol tartrate (Betaloc) :**
   Oral : 50, 100 mg tablets.
   Dose : 100-200 mg/day once in a day or divided doses.

3. **Acebutolol hydrochloride (Sectrol-200) :**
   Oral : 200 mg tablets.
   Dose : 200 mg twice in a day in the treatment of angina.

4. **Bisoprolol fumarate (Concor) :**
   Oral : 5 mg tablets.
   Dose : 5 mg once in a day in hypertension. Maximum dose 10 mg/day.

5. **Esmolol hydrochloride :**
   Parenteral : 10 mg/mL.
   Mainly used during surgery to control supraventricular arrhythmias (including atrial flutter, atrial fibrillation, sinus tachycardia), tachycardia and hypertension.

Non-selective Beta-receptor blockers

1. **Labetalol hydrochloride (Normadate) :**
   Oral : 50, 100, 200 mg tablets.
   Dose : 50 mg twice in a day with food in hypertension.

2. **Pindolol (Visken) :**
   Oral : 10 mg tablets.
   Dose : 10-30 mg/day in the treatment of hypertension.

3. **Propranolol hydrochloride (Inderal) :**
   Oral : 10, 20, 40, 60, 90 mg tablets.
   Solution : 4, 8 mg/mL.
   Injection : 1 mg/mL.
   Oral sustained release (Inderal LA) : 80, 120, 160 mg cap.
   Dose : 10-40 mg 3-4 times daily.
   Used in hypertension and thyrotoxicosis.

4. **Sotalol hydrochloride (Sotagard) :**
   Oral : 40 mg tablets.
   Dose : 80-160 mg/day used in cardiac arrhythmias.

Calcium channel blockers

1. **Amlodipine besylate (Amcard, Amdepin, Amlodac, Amlogard, Amlong, Amprez, Angiguard) :**
   Oral : 2.5, 5, 10 mg tablets.
   Dose : 5-10 mg once in a day in the treatment of hypertension.

2. **Benidipine (Caritec) :**
   Oral : 4, 8 mg Film coated tablets.
   Dose : 4 mg once in a day in hypertension.

3. **Diltiazem (Dicard, Dilcal, Dilcardia, Dilgard, Dilgina, Diltine, Dizem) :**
   Oral : 30, 60 mg tablets.
   90, 120 mg sustained release tablets.
   Dose : 30 mg four times in a day.
   90 mg twice in a day.
   Used in mild to moderate hypertension and in angina.

4. **Felodipine (Felogard, Plendil) :**
   Oral : 2.5, 5, 10 mg sustained release tablets.
   Dose : 5 mg once in a day in the treatment of mild to moderate hypertension.

5. **Lacidipine (Sinopil) :**
   Oral : 2, 4 mg tablets.
   Dose : Adults 4 mg/day once daily preferably in the morning.
   Elderly patient 2 mg/day.
   Used in the treatment of hypertension.

6. **Nifedipine (Nicardia, Nifelat) :**
   Oral : 10, 20, 30 mg tablets.
   Dose : 10-20 mg twice in a day in hypertension.

7. **Nitrendipine (Nitrepin) :**
   Oral : 10, 20 mg tablets.
   Dose : 5-20 mg once in a day in mild to moderate hypertension.

8. **Verapamil hydrochloride (Calaptin) :**
   Oral : 40, 80 mg dragees.
   Dose : 40-80 mg thrice in a day in angina and arrhythmias.
   Injection : 5 mg/2 mL.
   In acute coronary spasm 1.5 mg/kg/day slow intravenous infusion with ECG monitoring.

EXPERIMENT 3

Identification of unknown sample of drug using isolated frog heart

AIM

To find out the effect and mechanism(s) of action of the given sample of drug using isolated frog heart.

PRINCIPLE

Heart is supplied by autonomic nervous system. Beta-receptor agonists like adrenaline, isoprenaline etc. act on the beta-receptors present in the heart and increase the heart rate and amplitude. Beta-receptor blocking agents like propranolol, atenolol antagonise the actions of beta-agonists. Muscarinic agonists (acetylcholine, carbachol, muscarine etc.) act on the muscarinic receptors present in the heart and decrease the heart rate and amplitude and in higher doses stop the heart beat during diastolic phase. Muscarinic antagonists like atropine, homatropine antagonise the action of muscarinic agonists. Potassium chloride excess concentration in the Frog Ringer solution stops the heart beat during diastolic phase. Excess calcium ions in the perfusion medium stop the heart beat during systolic phase. Inorganic ions like potassium and calcium act on the cardiac muscle through the non-receptor mechanism of action.

EQUIPMENTS AND OTHER MATERIALS REQUIRED

INCO kymograph, starling heart lever, L-stand, T-rod, X-blocks, Syme's cannula, screw clip, mariotte bottle, rubber tubes, tuberculine syringe, 26 No. needle, surgical instruments.

Animal

Frog.

Physiological solution required

Frog ringer solution.

Drug solutions required

Adrenaline hydrochloride 10 microgram per ml in distilled water.

Acetylcholine hydrochloride 10 microgram per mL in distilled water.

Potassium chloride 4% in distilled water.

Calcium chloride 4% in distilled water.

Propranolol hydrochloride 100 microgram per mL in distilled water.

Atropine sulphate 100 microgram per mL in distilled water.

Verapamil 1 microgram per ml.

PROCEDURE

1. Set up the isolated heart experiment as described in experiment No. 2 (perform step 1 to step 16 of experiment No. 2).
2. Inject 0.05 ml of the given test solution into Syme's cannula. Immediately switch on the kymograph and record the effect of test sample for 2 minutes period. If the sample does not exhibit any significant change of the heart rate or amplitude, then gradually increase the dose of test sample.
3. Proceed further depending upon the type of response produced by test sample.

   For example :

   A. If the test sample produces an increase in heart rate and amplitude, then administer a beta-receptor blocking agent like propanolol hydrochloride 100 µg/ml (Dose 0.5 to 1 ml) and repeat the dose of the test sample. If the sample fails to produce an increase in heart rate and amplitude after the administration of a beta-blocker, it indicates that the given test sample is a beta-receptor agonist.

   B. If the test sample causes a decrease in heart rate and amplitude, then administer a muscarinic blocking agent like atropine sulphate 100 µg/ml (Dose 0.5 to 1 ml) and repeat the administration of the test sample. If the test sample fails to produce a decrease in heart rate and amplitude after the administration of muscarinic blocker, it indicates that the test sample is a muscarinic agonist. After atropinization, if the test sample produces diastolic block it indicates that the test sample is potassium chloride.

   C. If the test sample does not produce any significant change of heart rate or amplitude it indicates that the test sample is an antagonist or water for injection. Then give 1 ml of test sample and after 1 minute administer same dose of adrenaline used for recording standard response. If the response of adrenaline is antagonised by the test sample, it indicates that the given sample is a beta-receptor antagonist.

D. If the test sample antagonises the effect of muscarinic agonist, then the given sample is a muscarinic antagonist.

E. If the test sample does not alter the responses of adrenaline, acetylcholine, potassium chloride or calcium chloride it indicates that the given sample is water for injection or frog Ringer solution.

F. If the test sample produces stoppage of heart beat during systolic phase, it indicates that the given sample contain calcium ions. Administer a calcium channel blocker like verapamil and repeat the dose of test sample. Therefore, by using selective agonists and antagonists it is possible to screen a large number of drugs which act on the cardiovascular system.

Things to remember

Whenever experiments are set up to identify the effect and mechanism of action of the given sample,the following steps must be followed (to avoid error in the identification of drugs) :

1. First record the effect of standard drugs (like adrenaline, acetylcholine, calcium chloride, potassium chloride) i.e. Agonist only.

2. After the administration of standard drugs administer the test drug.

EXPERIMENT 4

Identification of unknown sample of drug using perfused frog heart

AIM

To find out the effect and mechanism(s) of action of the given sample of drug using perfused frog heart.

PRINCIPLE

Same as Experiment No. 3.

EQUIPMENTS AND OTHER MATERIALS REQUIRED

ICNO kymograph, starling heart lever, L-stand, T-rod, X-blocks, Venous cannula, screw clip, mariotte bottle, rubber tubes, tuberculine syringe, 26 or 29 No. needle, surgical instruments.

Animal

Frog.

Physiological solution required

Frog Ringer solution.

Drug solutions required

Adrenaline hydrochloride 10 microgram/mL.

Acetylcholine hydrochloride 10 microgram/mL.

Potassium chloride 4% in distilled water.

Calcium chloride 4% in distilled water.

Propranolol hydrochloride 100 microgram/mL in distilled water.

Atropine sulphate 100 microgram/mL in distilled water.

Verapamil 1 microgram/mL.

PROCEDURE

1. Set up the assembly for the above mentioned experiment.
2. Pith a frog by passing a needle through the occipito-atlantic

junction between the brain and spinal cord. The stretching out of limbs indicate that the pithing is proper.

3. Place the frog in a tray with the ventral side facing up.

4. Make an incision of the skin longitudinally and then expose the rectus muscle.

5. Make incision around the rectus muscle without damaging the anterior abdominal vein.

6. Expose the heart after cutting the sternum.

7. Remove the pericardial membrane.

8. Tie one side of the aorta.

9. Put a knot around the inferior venacava then make a small cut for cannulation.

10. After cannulation with venous cannula, cut the other side of the aorta.

11. Place the frog on a frog board and perfuse the heart with frog Ringer solution. Adjust the flow of the frog Ringer's solution through the venous cannula.

12. Place a heart-clip on the apex of the heart and connect it to a starling heart lever.

13. Record the normal heart beat on a smoked drum.

14. Inject 0.05-0.1 ml of adrenaline solution into the perfusion rubber tube using 26 or 29 No. needle. Immediately switch on the kymograph and record the effect of adrenaline for 2 minutes period. After 2 minutes switch off the kymograph till the heart beat and amplitude comes to normal and observe the onset and duration of action of adrenaline.

15. Inject 0.05-0.1 ml of acetylcholine into the perfusion rubber tube. Immediately switch on the kymograph and record the effect of acetylcholine for 2 minutes. After 2 minutes switch off the kymograph till the heart beat and amplitude comes to normal. Observe the onset and duration of action of acetylcholine.

16. Inject 0.1 ml of potassium chloride solution into the perfusion tube. Immediately switch on the kymograph and record the effect of potassium chloride for 2 minutes period. After 2 minutes switch off the kymograph till the heart beat and amplitude comes to normal. Observe the onset and duration of action of potassium chloride.

17. Inject 0.1 to 0.4 ml of calcium chloride solution into the perfusion

tube. Immediately switch on the kymograph and record the effect of calcium chloride for 2 minutes period. After 2 minutes switch off the kymograph till the heart rate and amplitude comes to normal. Observe the onset and duration of action of calcium chloride.

18. Inject 0.05 ml of the given test solution into the perfusion tube. Immediately switch on the kymograph and record the effect of test sample for 2 minutes period. If the sample does not exhibit any change of the heart rate or amplitude, then gradually increase the dose of test sample.

19. Proceed further depending upon the type of response produced by the test sample.

For Example :

A. If the test sample produces an increase in heart rate and amplitude, then administer a beta-receptor blocking agent like propranolol hydrochloride 100 µg/ml (dose 0.5-1 ml) and repeat the dose of the test sample. If the sample fails to produce an increase in heart rate and amplitude after the administration of a beta-blocker, it indicates that the given test sample is a beta-receptor agonist.

B. If the test sample causes a decrease in heart rate and amplitude, wait till the heart rate and amplitude comes to normal, then administer a muscarinic blocking agent like atropine sulphate 100 µg/ml (dose 0.5 to 1 ml) and repeat the administration of the test sample. If the test sample fails to produce a decrease in heart rate and amplitude after the administration of muscarinic blocker, it indicates that the test sample is a muscarinic agonist. After atropinization, if the test sample produces diastolic block it indicates that the test sample is potassium chloride.

C. If the test sample does not produce any significant change of heart rate or amplitude, it indicates that the test sample is an antagonist or water for injection. Then give 1 ml of the test sample and after one minute administer same dose of adrenaline used for recording standard response. If the response of adrenaline is antagonised by the test sample it indicates that the given sample is a beta-receptor antagonist.

D. If the test sample antagonises the effect of muscarinic agonist, then the given sample is a muscarinic antagonist.

E. If the test sample does not alter the responses of adrenaline, acetylcholine, potassium chloride or calcium chloride, it indicates the given sample is water for injection or frog Ringer solution.

F. If the test sample produces stoppage of heart beat during systolic phase, it indicates that the given sample contain calcium ions. Administer a calcium channel blocker like verapamil (0.1 ml 1 µg/ml) and after 1 minute repeat the dose the test sample.

Therefore, by using selective agonists and antagonists it is possible to screen a large number of drugs which act on the cardiovascular system.

EXPERIMENT 5

Effect of vasoconstrictors and vasodilators on blood vessels of frog

AIM

To study the effect of nor-adrenaline, acetylcholine, histamine, nitroprusside, sodium nitrite, verapamil hydrochloride and pinacidil on blood vessels of frog.

PRINCIPLE

Nor-adrenaline acts on alpha-1 receptors and produces vasoconstriction. Acetylcholine acts on muscarinic receptors and produces vasodilatation. Histamine acts on H_1 and H_2 receptors and produces vasodilatation. Nitroprusside and sodium nitrite release nitric oxide and cause vasodilatation. Verapamil is a calcium channel blocker, because of this property verapamil produces vasodilatation. Pinacidil is a potassium channel opener, hence it produces vasodilatation.

EQUIPMENTS AND OTHER MATERIALS REQUIRED

Mariotte bottle, Rubber tubes, Frog board, Screw clip, Venous cannula.

Animal

Frog (bigger size).

Physiological solution required

Frog Ringer solution.

Drug solutions required

1. Nor-adrenaline acid tartrate 4 microgram/ml.
2. Acetylcholine hydrochloride 10 microgram/mL.
3. Histamine hydrochloride 10 microgram/mL.
4. Nitroprusside 10 microgram/mL.
5. Sodium nitrite one per cent.
6. Verapamil hydrochloride 5 microgram/mL.
7. Pinacidil 1 microgram/mL.

PROCEDURE

1. Set up the assembly for the above experiment.
2. Pith a frog and expose the heart after removing the pericardial membrane.
3. Adjust the flow of the Ringer solution from the Mariotte bottle using screw clip and perfusion tube.
4. Cannulate left branch of aorta using venous cannula and perfuse with frog Ringer solution.
5. Cannulate the inferior vena cava in the opposite direction, so that the perfusate comes out through the inferior vena-cava.
6. Tie the other branch of the aorta.
7. When the Frog Ringer solution coming out of inferior vena-cava becomes clear, count the number of drops per minute.
8. Inject 0.1 ml of nor-adrenaline into the perfusion tube and count the number of drops coming out of the inferior vena-cava. Observe the onset and duration of action of nor-adrenaline.
9. Record the responses of other drugs in similar way.

OBSERVATIONS AND CONCLUSION

1. Nor-adrenaline reduced the number of drops coming out of the inferior vena cava which indicates that nor-adrenaline is a vasoconstrictor.
2. Acetylcholine, histamine hydrochloride, nitroprusside, sodium nitrite, verapamil hydrochloride and pinacidil increased the number of drops coming out of the inferior vena cava which indicates that these drugs produce a vasodilatory effect.

Things to remember

The following vasoconstrictors and vasodilators are available for clinical uses.

I. Vasoconstrictors

1. **Ephedrine hydrochloride :**

   Dose : 3-6 mg tablets. 3 mg/mL slow intravenous infusion in hypotension.

2. **Metaraminol :**

   Dose : 15-100 mg in 500 ml slow intravenous infusion.

3. **Methoxamine hydrochloride :**
   Dose : 5-10 mg slow intravenous infusion.
4. **Nor-adrenaline acid tartrate :**
   Dose : 8 µg/mL 2-3 mL/minute intravenous infusion.
5. **Phenylephrine hydrochloride :**
   Dose : 100-500 microgram slow intravenous infusion.

II. Vasodilators

The following nitrates are used in the treatment of angina :

1. **Erythrityl tetranitrate (Cardilate) :**
   Oral : 5, 15 mg tablets.
   Dose : 5-10 mg sublingually or orally 3 to 4 times daily.
2. **Isosorbide mononitrate (Angicor, Anginex, Imdur) :**
   Oral : 10, 20, 40, 60 mg tablets.
   Dose : 10-20 mg 2-3 times daily.
3. **Glyceryltrinitrate (Angised, Angispan TR, Millisrol, Myonit, Myovin, Nitroglycerin, Nitrocontin, Nitroderm, Nitroject) :**
   Oral : 0.5, 2.6, 6.4 mg tablets. 2.5, 6.5 mg capsules.
   Injection : 5 mg/mL.
   Ointment : 2%.
   Dose : Sublingually 0.5 to 1 mg as required.
   By mouth 2.6-6.4 mg 2-3 times daily.
   Transdermal 5-10 mg/24 hours.
4. **Isosorbide dinitrate (Cardicap, Ditrate, Isomack retard, Isodril, Sorbicap, Sorbitrate) :**
   Oral : 5, 10 mg tablets. 20, 40 mg sustained release tablets.
   Dose : Sublingually 5-10 mg.
   By mouth 30-120 mg/day.
5. **Pentaerythritol tetranitrate (Peritrate) :**
   Oral : 10 mg tablets,
   80 mg sustained release tablets.
   Dose : 30 mg 3-4 times daily.
   80 mg 2 times daily.

Calcium channel blockers

Name of the calcium channel blockers used in clinical practice are mentioned in experiment No. 3.

Potassium channel openers

Following potassium channel openers are used as vasodilators.

1. Pinacidil
2. Nicorandil.

EXPERIMENT 6

Effect of cardiac glycoside (Digoxin/Digitoxin) on frog heart

AIM

To study the cardiotonic effect of digoxin on isolated frog heart.

PRINCIPLE

Digoxin is a cardiac glycoside. It is one of the constituents present in *Digitalis purpurea.* Digoxin inhibits the Na^+ K+ ATPase enzyme and increases the intracellular calcium in the ventricle. Thus digoxin increases the force of contraction of the heart. Therefore, digoxin is used in the treatment of congestive heart failure. Perfusion of frog heart with frog Ringer solution containing low calcium concentration (0.275 mM) produces decrease in the heart rate. Administration of digoxin improves the force of contraction of the hypodynamic heart.

EQUIPMENTS AND OTHER MATERIALS REQUIRED

INCO kymograph, starling heart lever, L-stand, T-rod, X-blocks, Syme's cannula, Screw clip, Mariotte bottle, rubber tubes, Tuberculine syringe, 26 No. needle, Surgical instruments.

Animal

Frog.

Physiological solutions required

1. Frog Ringer solution containing 1.1 mM calcium chloride.
2. Frog Ringer solution containing 0.275 mM calcium chloride.

Drug solutions required

Digoxin 50 microgram/mL.
Digitoxin 50 microgram/mL.

PROCEDURE

1. Set up the assembly for the above mentioned experiment as shown below :

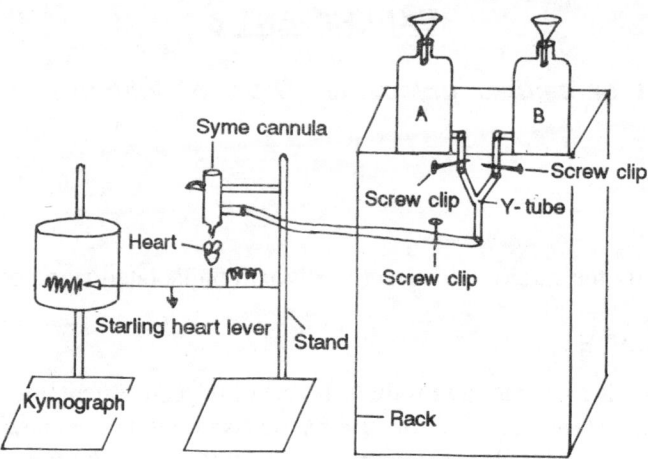

Fig. Ex. 6.1. Set up for the isolated frog heart to study the effect of digoxin. A. Frog Ringer solution containing 1.1 mM calcium chloride. B. Frog Ringer solution containing 0.275 mM calcium chloride.

2. Fill the first Mariottle bottle (marked A) with frog Ringer solution containing 1.1 mM calcium chloride.

3. Adjust the flow of the frog Ringer solution from Mariottle bottle A using screw clip.

4. Pith a frog by passing a needle through the occipito-atlantic junction between the brain and the spinal cord. The stretching out of limbs indicate that the pithing is proper.

5. Place the frog in a tray with the ventral side facing up.

6. Make an incision of the skin longitudinally and then expose the rectus muscle.

7. Make incision around the rectus muscle without damaging anterior abdominal vein.

8. Expose the heart after cutting the sternum.

9. Remove the pericardial membrane.

10. Tie one side of the aorta.

11. Put a knot around the inferior vena cava then make a small 'v' shaped cut for cannulation.

12. After cannulation with Syme's cannula, cut the other side of the aorta and isolate the heart from the body and perfuse with frog Ringer solution containing 1.1 mM of calcium chloride.

13. Place a heart-clip on the apex of the ventricle and connect it to a starling heart lever.

14. Record the normal heart beat on a smoked drum.
15. Fill the second Mariotte bottle (marked B) with frog Ringer solution containing 0.275 mM calcium chloride.
16. Block the flow of frog Ringer solution from Mariotte bottle A.
17. Perfuse the heart with frog Ringer solution from Mariottle bottle B.
18. Record the reduction in the force of contraction of the heart on a smoked drum.
19. Inject different doses of digoxin/digitoxin (50, 100 microgram) into the Syme's cannula and record the force of contraction.
20. Inject 1000 microgram of digoxin and record the response.
21. Block the flow of frog Ringer solution from Mariottle bottle B.
22. Perfuse the heart with frog Ringer solution from Mariottle bottle A and record the heart beat.

OBSERVATION AND CONCLUSION

1. When the frog heart is perfused with frog Ringer solution containing 1.1 mM calcium chloride, the heart rate and force of contraction are normal.

2. When the frog heart is perfused with frog Ringer solution containing 0.275 mM calcium chloride the force of contraction is reduced. Administration of cardiac glucoside (digoxin/digitoxin) increased the force of contraction.

3. Digoxin at low doses improves the efficiency of hypodynamic heart because it inhibits $Na^+K^+ATPase$ and increases intracellular calcium in the ventricle.

4. Very high dose (toxic dose) of digoxin stops the heart beat in systolic phase, because of excess calcium concentration in the ventricle.

Things to remember

Congestive Heart Failure is a syndrome characterized by tachycardia, pulmonary oedema and cardiomegaly, which occurs due to failure of the heart to meet the demands of the body. The efficiency of cardiac output in Congestive Heart Failure is below the normal range. Cardiac glycosides like digoxin and digitoxin are used in congestive heart failure. The following cardiac glycosides are available for clinical uses.

1. **Digitoxin (Crystodigin) :**
   Oral : 0.05, 0.1, 0.15, 0.2 mg tablets.
   Dose : Adult : 50-100 micrograms/day.

2. **Digoxin (Lanoxin) :**
   Oral : 0.25, 0.5 mg tablets; Elixir 0.05 mg/mL.
   Dose : Adults and children above 10 years.
   Initial Dose : 0.25-1.5 mg/day.
   Maintenance Dose : 0.0625-0.5 mg/day.
   Elderly patient : 0.0125 mg/day.
   Parenteral : 0.5 mg/2 mL injection.

Contraindications : Ventricular arrhythmias, diastolic failure, heart block and obstructive cardiac myopathy.

Experiments on Skeletal Muscle

EXPERIMENT 7

Effect of acetylcholine on rectus abdominis muscle of frog.

AIM

(i) To study the action of acetylcholine on rectus abdominis muscle.

(ii) Recording of concentration response curve of acetylcholine and determination of pD_2 value.

PRINCIPLE

Frog rectus abdominis muscle is a voluntary muscle. At the neuromuscular junction, a nerve impulse liberates acetylcholine from the nerve ending into the cleft between muscle and nerve fibre. This acetylcholine causes a depolarization of the muscle fibre which in turn sets off a muscle action potential, and contraction of the muscle fibre. The muscle fibres of lower species like frog are multiply innervated and hence nerve stimulation causes persistent depolarization and a prolonged slow contraction of the muscle. Local administration of acetylcholine also produces similar effect. Frog rectus abdominus muscle contains nicotinic (N_2) receptors. Acetylcholine acts as an agonist.

EQUIPMENTS REQUIRED

Student Kymograph, Studentorganbath, aeration tube, aerator, aeration tube holder, frontal writing lever, lever holder, screw clip, haemostatic forceps, mariotte bottle, rubber tubes, tuberculine syringe, 26 No. needle, pithing needle, scissor, forceps.

Animal required : Frog.

Physiological solution required

Frog Ringer solution.

Drug solution required

Acetylcholine 100 micrograms per ml.

PROCEDURE

1. Set up the assembly for the above mentioned experiment.
2. Pith a frog by passing a needle through the occipito-atlantic junction between the brain and the spinal cord. The stretching out of the limbs indicate that the pithing is proper.
3. Place the frog in a tray with the ventral side facing up.
4. Pick up the skin of abdomen with the help of forceps and make-proper incision to expose the abdomen.
5. Cut along the margin of the rectus abdominis muscle and then make a transverse cut through the sternum just above the base.
6. Free the rectus abdominus muscle from the anterior abdominal vein.
7. Lift the muscle gently and divide the muscle longitudinally.
8. Tie a long thread on the upper side of the rectus muscle and a short thread on the lower side of the rectus abdominus muscle.
9. Transfer the muscle to a petri-dish containing frog Ringer solution.
10. Tie the short thread to the hook of the aeration tube and place the rectus muscle in the inner organ bath containing frog ringer solution.
11. Tie the long thread to a frontal writing lever. The load on the lever should be 1 gram. The magnification should be between 5-7 times.
12. Stabilize the rectus muscle for 55 minutes period.
13. During the stabilization period replace the frog ringer solution in the inner organ bath at an interval of 5 minutes.
14. After stabilization for a period of 55 minutes, switch on the Kymograph and record the normal tracing for a period of 30 seconds. At the end of 30 seconds period inject 0.1 ml of acetylcholine solution into the inner organ bath and record the tracings for a period of 90 seconds (Drug contact time). At the end of 90 seconds switch off the Kymograph and give 3-4 washings of rectus muscle with frog ringer solution.
15. Inject 0.1 ml of acetylcholine solution into the inner organ bath once again and record the response for 90 seconds.

16. If two equipotent responses are observed with similar doses of acetylcholine, then record the responses of acetylcholine with higher doses (0.2, 0.4, 0.8 and 1 ml) as shown below.

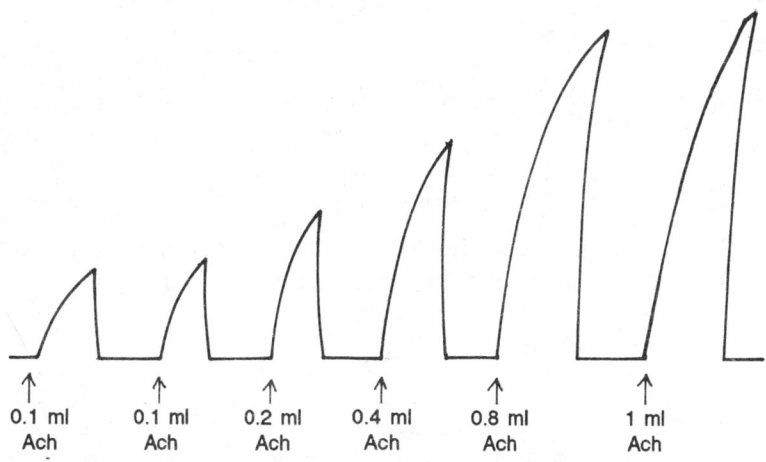

↑	↑	↑	↑	↑	↑
0.1 ml	0.1 ml	0.2 ml	0.4 ml	0.8 ml	1 ml
Ach	Ach	Ach	Ach	Ach	Ach

17. After fixing the graph measure the height of contraction of the response produced by each dose of acetylcholine and find out the dose which produces maximal response.

S.No.	Dose of acetylcholine in ml	Log dose of Acetylcholine	Height of contraction (Response) in mm
1.	0.1	T.0000	20
2.	0.1	T.0000	20
3.	0.2	T.3010	40
4.	0.4	T.6021	78
5.	0.8	T.9031	90
6.	1	0.0000	91

18. Plot a graph showing dose of acetylcholine on X-axis and response on Y-axis.

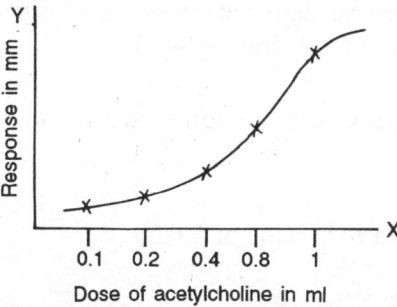

19. Plot another graph showing log dose of acetylcholine on X-axis and response on Y-axis.

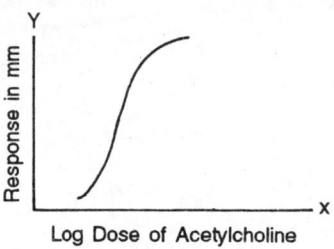

Log Dose of Acetylcholine

20. Plot a third graph showing log molar concentration of acetylcholine on X-axis and percentage response on Y axis.

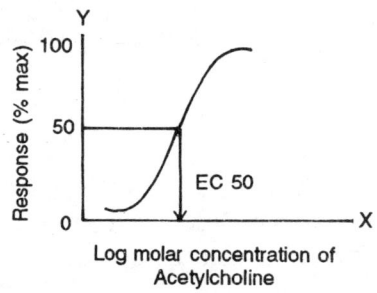

Log molar concentration of
Acetylcholine

21. From the graph find out the EC $_{50}$.

22. From the EC_{50} value find out the pD_2 value.

For example :

If the $EC_{50} = 9.5 \times 10^{-7}$

$$(M \times 10^{-n})$$

Then $pD_2 = n - \log m$

$$= 7 - \log 9.5$$

$$= 7 - 0.98$$

$$= 6.02.$$

Therefore, one can define pD_2 value as the negative log of molar concentration of the drug exhibiting half of the maximal response.

pD_2 value gives us information about the affinity of a drug for a particular receptor.

For example :

Drug A has a pD_2 value of 5.02.

Drug B has a pD_2 value of 6.02.

Drug C has a pD_2 value of 7.

This indicates that drug C is the most potent drug.

OBSERVATIONS AND CONCLUSION

1. Acetylcholine produced a dose-dependent contraction effect on frog rectus abdominis muscle.

2. A graph plotted with a linear concentration scale shows non-sigmoid dose-response curve.

3. A graph plotted with a logarithmic concentration scale shows a sigmoid dose-response curve.

4. Determination of pD_2 value is useful to find out the affinity of a drug for a particular receptor.

EXPERIMENT 8

Biotransformation of acetylcholine by cholinesterase enzyme

AIM

To demonstrate the destruction of acetylcholine by plasma cholinesterase enzyme.

PRINCIPLE

Cholinesterase enzymes cause the hydrolysis of acetylcholine. Two types of cholinesterase are present in the body. They are acetylcholinesterase and butyrylcholine-esterase.

EQUIPMENTS REQUIRED

Same as experiment No. 7.

Animal required

Frog.

Physiological solution required

Frog Ringer solution.

Drug solution required

Acetylcholine 100 micrograms per ml.

Serum/plasma 1 mL.

PROCEDURE

1. Follow the step No. 1 to 16 of experiment No. 7.
2. After recording the concentration response curve of acetylcholine, select a dose of acetylcholine which gives about 50% of the maximum response.
3. Take two test tubes and number them.

   In test tube No. 1, take 0.2 ml of acetylcholine (EC_{50} dose) and 0.2 ml of Ringer solution and incubate at 37°C for 5 minutes. Then add the whole content into the inner organ bath and record the response for 90 seconds. Wash the preparation till it comes to normal.

4. In test tube No. 2 take 0.2 ml of acetylcholine (EC_{50} dose) and 0.2 ml of serum and incubate at 37°C for 5 minutes. Then add the whole content into the inner organ bath and record the response for 90 seconds. Wash the preparation till it comes to normal.

OBSERVATIONS AND CONCLUSION

1. The solution in test tube No. 1 produces response identical to the response produced by EC_{50} dose of acetylcholine.

2. The solution in test tube No. 2 produced response less than that produced by EC_{50} dose of acetylcholine, because cholinesterase present in the serum/plasma caused the hydrolysis of acetylcholine and reduced its concentration.

Things to remember

Butyrylcholinesterase (pseudocholinesterase) present in the plasma hydrolyses butyrylcholine, acetylcholine, succinylcholine, procaine, propanidid etc.

Succinylcholine chloride (Suxamethonium chloride) (Midarine, Scoline) is used as a short acting muscle relaxant. In patients with atypical cholinesterase (Abnormal cholinesterase), the duration of action of succinylcholine lasts for an hour, because succinylcholine and atypical cholinesterase do not combine readily, hence, succinylcholine will not be hydrolysed rapidly in such patients. Therefore, such patients show prolonged apnea. The in vitro studies also show high Km value.

Dibucaine number

Dibucaine is a local anaesthetic not used widely due to its toxicity.

Dibucaine is an inhibitor of cholinesterase enzymes.

Dibucaine inhibits the atypical cholinesterase enzyme less than the normal cholinesterase enzyme.

Dibucaine number can be defined as the measure of the percentage inhibition of plasma cholinesterase by Dibucaine at a concentration of 10^{-6} mol/litre. Therefore, the plasma of patients with atypical cholinesterase or abnormal cholinesterase show a low dibucaine number.

EXPERIMENT 9

Potentiation of the action of acetylcholine by anticholinesterase agents

AIM

To demonstrate the potentiation of the action of acetylcholine by anticholinesterase agents like neostigmine or physostigmine.

PRINCIPLE

Cholinesterase is an enzyme. It is inhibited by anticholinesterase agents. There are two types of anticholinesterase agents. Reversible inhibitors of cholinesterase are neostigmine and physostigmine. Irreversible inhibitors are organophosphorus compounds like parathion, malathion etc. Anticholinesterase agents potentiate the action of acetylcholine at the neuromuscular junction. The term potentiation refers to the administration of two drugs simultaneously which produce a response greater than the sum of their independent actions.

EQUIPMENTS REQUIRED

Same as experiment No. 7.

Physiological solution required

Frog Ringer solution.

Animal

Frog.

Drug solution required

Acetylcholine 100 μg/mL.
Neostigmine 100 μg/ml.
Physostigmine 100 μg/ml.

PROCEDURE

1. Follow the steps 1 to 16 of the experiment No. 7.
2. Add 0.5 ml of neostigmine (50 μg) into the inner organ bath. Allow it to act for 5 minutes. Then inject the lowest dose of

acetylcholine and record the response for 90 seconds. Wash the rectus muscle with frog Ringer solution till the writing point of the frontal writing lever comes to the base line.

3. Repeat the above step with higher doses of acetylcholine and record a concentration Response Curve of acetylcholine in the presence of neostigmine.

4. Plot a graph showing log dose of acetylcholine on X-axis and response on Y-axis in the absence of neostigmine (see Experiment No. 7).

5. In the above graph also show the log dose of acetylcholine on X-axis and response on Y-axis in the presence of neostigmine as shown below :

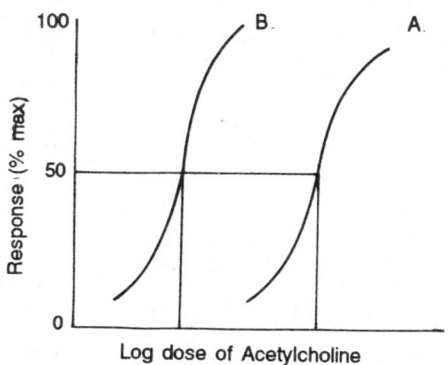

A = Acetylcholine B = Neostigmine + Acetylcholine

From the above graph calculate the dose ratio. In the presence of neostigmine, the agonist (Acetylcholine) log concentration effect curve is shifted to the **left** without change in the slope or maximum response, the extent of shift being a measure of the dose-ratio of acetylcholine.

Dose ratio of acetylcholine = $\dfrac{EC_{50} \text{ of Acetylcholine in the presence of neostigmine}}{EC_{50} \text{ of acetylcholine in the absence of neostigmine}}$

OBSERVATIONS AND CONCLUSION

The effect of acetylcholine is potentiated in the presence of neostigmine. Hence, CRC of acetylcholine is shifted towards left in the presence of neostigmine.

Things to remember

Myasthenia gravis is a neuromuscular disorder. Neostigmine is clinically used in this disorder. The following preparations are available for clinical use :

1. **Neostigmine bromide (Tilstigmin) :**

   Oral : 15 mg tablets.

   Dose : Neonate : 1-5 mg every 4 hrs.

   Child : 1-6 years 7.5 mg every 4 hours.

   Adult : 60-90 mg in divided doses.

2. **Neostigmine methylsulphate (Myostigmin) :**

   Parenteral : 0.5, 2.5, 5 mg/mL, sc, i.m.

   Neonate : 50-250 micrograms per 4 hours.

   Child : 200-500 micrograms per 4 hours.

   Adult : 1-2.5 mg as required.

EXPERIMENT 10

Pharmacological antagonism

AIM

(a) To show the agonistic effect of acetylcholine on the frog rectus abdominis muscle and its antagonism by neuromuscular blocking agents (Anti-deploraising agents) like pancuronium or d-tubocurarine or gallamine.

(b) Determination of dose-ratio and pA_2 value.

PRINCIPLE

Antagonism refers to the opposing actions of two drugs on the same physiological system. The opposing actions of an agonist and an antagonist at specific receptor sites leads to Pharmacological antagonism. The principle of Pharmacological antagonism is useful in the treatment of drug poisoning. Acetylcholine acts as an agonist at the nicotinic receptor sites and produces contraction effect. This effect is blocked by nicotinic receptor antagonists like pancuronium or d-tubocurarine or gallamine.

EQUIPMENTS AND OTHER MATERIALS REQUIRED

Same as Experiment No. 7.

Animal required

Frog.

Physiological solution required

Frog Ringer solution.

Drug solutions used

Acetylcholine : 100 micrograms per ml.

Pancuronium : 100 nanograms per ml.

PROCEDURE

1. Follow steps 1 to 15 of the experiment No. 7.

2. If two equipotent responses are observed with similar doses of acetylcholine, then record a cumulative dose response curve of acetylcholine as shown below.

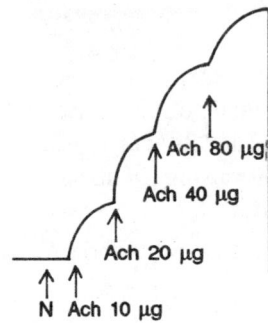

(Inject 0.1 ml of acetylcholine and record the response for 90 seconds, without washing the tissue then inject 0.2 ml (20 μg) of acetylcholine and record the response for 90 seconds. Similarly record the responses of acetylcholine with higher doses till the maximum response is observed).

3. Add pancuronium into the inner organ bath so that the final concentration is 1 nanogram/mL wait for five minutes, then record a cumulative dose response graph of acetylcholine in presence of pancuronium. The doses of acetylcholine have to be increased inorder to get the maximum response of acetylcholine in presence of an antagonist.

4. Give washing several times with Frog Ringer solution and record the cumulative dose response graph of acetylcholine.

5. Add pancuronium solution into the inner organ bath so that the final concentration is 2 ng/mL. Then record a cumulative dose response graph of acetylcholine in presence of pancuronium.

6. Give washings till the tissue recovers from the effect of pancuronium and record a cumulative dose response graph of acetylcholine.

7. Add pancuronium into the inner organ bath so that the final concentration is 4 ng/mL. Then record the cumulative dose response graph of acetylcholine in presence of pancuronium.

8. From the graph obtained plot log dose response curves of acetylcholine in absence and in presence of pancuronium as shown below.

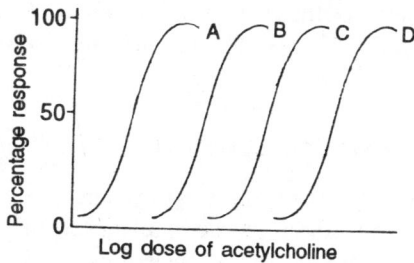

A = Cumulative dose response curve of acetylcholine
B = Cumulative dose response curve of acetylcholine in presence of pancuronium 1 ng/mL.
C = Cumulative dose response curve of acetylcholine in presence of pancuronum 2 ng/mL.
D = Cumulative dose response curve of acetylcholine in presence of pancuronium 4 ng/mL.

9. Find out the dose ratio from the graph.

$$\text{Dose Ratio (DR)} = \frac{EC_{50} \text{ of acetylcholine in presence of pancuronium}}{EC_{50} \text{ of acetylcholine in absence of pancuronium}}$$

10. Plot a graph showing log molar concentration of antagonist on X-axis and log (dose ratio-1) on Y-axis as shown below :

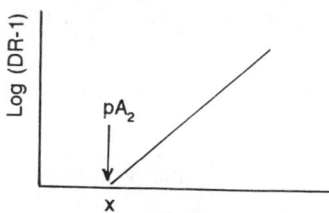

The log value obtained (x) is converted to negative log in order to get pA_2 value.

11. Make also a Schild plot from the graph as given below.

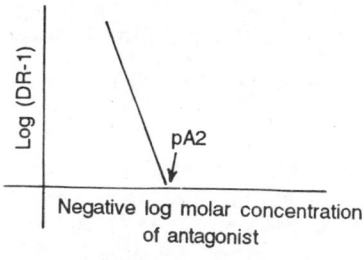

pA_2 value is the point where the line intersects the X-axis at the zero level of the Y axis. The higher value indicate high specificity.

OBSERVATIONS AND CONCLUSION

Acetylcholine is a nicotinic receptor agonist and hence produced a dose dependent contraction effect on skeletal muscle. Pancuronium is a nitocinic receptor antagonist. In presence of pancuronium, the concentration response curve of acetylcholine is shifted to right in a parallel manner which indicates that the type of antagonism is competitive.

Things to remember

The following drugs which act at the neuromuscular junction are used as muscle relaxant and are available for clinical uses during surgical anaesthesia.

I. Non-depolarising neuromuscular junction blockers

1. **Atracurium besylate (Tracrium) :**

   Parenteral : 10 mg/mL.

   Dose : 0.3-0.6 mg/kg by intravenous infusion.

2. **Pancuronium bromide (Neocuron, Panuron) :**

   Parenteral : 4 mg/2 mL.

   Dose : 40-100 micrograms per kg body weight given by I.V. route.

   Supplementary Dose : 10-20 micrograms per kg.

3. **Pipecuronium bromide (Arduan) :**

   Parenteral : 4 mg/mL.

   Dose : Initial 0.07-0.085 mg/kg by I.V. route.

   Incremental Dose : 0.01-0.015 mg/kg by I.V. route.

II. Depolarising neuromuscular junction blocker

Succinylcholine chloride (Midarine) :

Parenteral : 50 mg/mL.

Dose : 30-60 mg I.V. (Dose decided by the Physician according to the need of the patient).

EXPERIMENT 11

Identification of unknown sample of drug using frog rectus abdominis muscle

AIM

To find out the effect and mechanism of action of the given sample of drug using frog rectus abdominis muscle.

PRINCIPLE

Frog rectus abdominis muscle contains nicotinic N_2 receptors. Acetylcholine acts as an agonist. The effect of acetylcholine at the neuromuscular junction can be blocked by non-depolarising neuromuscular blocking agents like pancuronium, gallamine, d-tubocurarine etc. The effect of acetylcholine at the neuromuscular junction can be potentiated by anticholinesterase agents like physostigmine and neostigmine.

REQUIREMENTS

Equipments, animal, physiological solution and other materials required are similar to the requirement of Experiment No. 7.

Drug solutions required

Acetylcholine : 100 micrograms/mL.

Pancuronium : 100 nanograms/mL.

Neostigmine : 100 micrograms/mL.

PROCEDURE

1. Follow steps 1-16 of Experiment No. 7.

2. Administer a dose of acetylcholine which produces 50% of the maximal response (EC_{50} dose) and record the response for 90 seconds. Then give sufficient washings for recovery.

3. **Identification of an agonist :** Add 0.1 ml of test sample and record the response for 90 seconds. If the test sample produces contraction of the rectus muscle, it indicates that the sample is a nicotinic receptor agonist (If necessary the dose of the test sample can be increased).

4. Add 0.1 ml of pancuronium into the inner organ bath, wait for 5 minutes and then administer 0.1 ml of test sample. Failure of the test sample to produce a contraction effect in the presence of pancuronium indicates that the given sample is a nicotinic receptor agonist.

5. **Identification of an antagonist :** Add 0.1 ml of the test sample into the inner organ bath, if the sample fails to produce any response, it indicates that the given sample is an antagonist or Ringer solution or water for injection (if necessary the dose of the test sample can be increased upto 1 ml).

6. Add 0.1 ml of the test sample into the inner organ bath and allow it to act for 5 minutes. Then administer EC_{50} dose of acetylcholine in the presence of test sample and record the response of acetylcholine for 90 seconds. If the effect of EC_{50} dose of acetylcholine is reduced, it indicates the given test sample is an antagonist. If the test sample does not change the response of the EC_{50} dose of acetylcholine, it indicates that the given sample is Ringer solution or water for injection.

7. **Identification of cholinesterase inhibitors :** Add 0.1 ml of the test sample into the inner organ bath. After 5 minutes contact time add EC_{50} dose of acetylcholine and record the response for 90 seconds. If the response produced by EC_{50} dose of acetylcholine is increased, it indicates that the test sample is an anticholinesterase agent.

OBSERVATIONS AND CONCLUSION

1. Frog rectus abdominis muscle contains nicotinic receptors.

2. Acetylcholine acts as a nicotinic receptor agonist.

3. Pancuronium acts as a nicotinic receptor antagonist.

4. Neostigmine is an anticholinesterase agent.

5. Frog rectus abdominis muscle can be used for the identification of nicotinic receptor agonists, antagonists and anticholinesterase agents.

CHAPTER 5

Experiments on Smooth Muscle

EXPERIMENT 12

Effect of histamine, acetylcholine and barium chloride on guinea pig ileum

AIM

To study the effects of histamine, acetylcholine, barium chloride, chlorpheniramine, atropine and papaverine on guinea pig ileum.

PRINCIPLE

Guinea pig ileum is a smooth muscle. It is very sensitive to histamine (sensitivity is 0.005 microgram per ml). Histamine acts on H_1-receptors. Histamine acts as an agonist and produces contraction of guinea pig ileum. Histamine action on H_1-receptors is blocked by H_1-receptor antagonists like chlorpheniramine, mepyramine, astemizole, terfenadine etc. Acetylcholine acts as an agonist and produces contraction of guinea pig ileum. Acetylcholine action on muscarinic receptors is blocked by atropine and other para-sympatholytic drugs like homatropine, hyoscine etc. Barium chloride produces contraction of guinea pig ileum through non-receptor mechanism of action. It raises the intracellular calcium. Spasmogenic effects of barium chloride is blocked by spasmolytic agent like papaverine.

EQUIPMENTS REQUIRED

INCO Kymograph, student thermostatic organ bath, aeration tube, aerator, aeration tube holder, frontal writing lever, lever holder, screw clip, haemostatic forceps, mariotte bottle, rubber tubes, tuberculine syringe, 26 No. needle, suturing needle, scissor, forceps.

Animal required : Guinea pig.

Physiological solution required : Tyrode solution.

Drug solution required

Histamine hydrochloride 5 microgram per ml.

Acetyl choline 20 microgram per ml.

Barium chloride 4 per cent solution.

Chlorpheniramine maleate 1 microgram per ml.

Atropine sulphate 100 microgram per ml.

Papaverine hydrochloride 100 microgram per ml.

PROCEDURE

1. Fast a guinea pig for 12 hours period.
2. Set up the assembly for guinea pig ileum experiment.
3. Balance a frontal writing lever using plasticine and apply a tension of 500 mg.
4. Fill the outer jacket of the student organ bath with water.
5. Set the thermostat of the student organ bath at 37°C and put the switch on.
6. Fill the mariotte bottle with Tyrode solution and control the flow of Tyrode solution to the inner organ bath using haemostatic forceps.
7. When the temperature of the Tyrode solution reaches 37°C sacrify a guinea pig by giving a blow on the head and cutting the carotid artery.
8. Open the abdominal region and identify the ileo-caecal junction.
9. Remove a length of ileum and place it in a petridish containing Tyrode solution at 37°C and trim away the mesentery.
10. If the lumen of the ileum is not clear, wash it with Tyrode solution (37°C).
11. Cut a piece of ileum (approximately 3-4 cm) and using surgical suturing needle tie a thread at each end, taking care to see that the lumen of the ileum remained open.
12. Tie one end of the thread to the hook of the aeration tube and the other to a frontal writing lever.
13. Stabilize the tissue for 30 minutes period and aerate the guinea pig ileum in the inner organ bath with air.
14. Record the normal base line on the drum for 30 seconds. At the end of 30 second add 0.1 ml of histamine into the inner organ bath and record the response of the drug for 30 seconds. After recording the response for 30 seconds. Switch off the kymograph. Immediately open the out let of the inner organ bath and remove

the Tyrode's solution present in the inner-organ bath. Again fill the inner-organ bath with fresh Tyrode solution and keep it for 60 seconds Repeat the washing procedure 3-4 times or till the writing point of frontal lever comes to the base line. Then record the dose-dependent effect of histamine using higher doses. Give 3-4 wasings for recovery .

15. Record the responses of different doses of acetylcholine. Give 3-4 washings for recovery .
16. Record the responses of different doses of bariumchloride. Give 3-4 washing for recovery.
17. Add 0.1 ml of chlorpeniramine maleate into the innerorgan bath, allow it to act for 60 seconds then record the response of histamine in the presence of chlorpheniramine. Give 3-4 washings for recovery.
18. Add 0.1 ml of atropine sulphate solution into the inner organ bath, allow it to act for 60 seconds then record the response of acetylcholine in the presence of atropine sulphate. Give 3-4 washings for recovery.
19. Add 0.1 of papaverine hydrochloride solution into the inner organ bath, allow it to act for 60 seconnds then record the response of baruim chloride solution in the presence of papaverine hydrochloride. Give 3-4 washings for recovery.

OTHER EXERCISES

1. Record CRC of histamine and determine pD_2 value.
2. Record cumulative dose response curve of histamine in the absence and presence of H_1-receptor blocker and determine Dose Ratio and pA_2 value.
3. Record CRC of acetylcholine and determine pD_2 Value.
4. Record cumulative Dose Response Curve of acetylcholine in the absence and presence of atropine and determine dose ratio and pA_2 value.
5. Record CRC of acetylcholine in the absence and presence of papaverine and plot a line weaver and Burk plot graph and find out the type of antagonism.

Things to remember

Histamine is one of the autocoids released during allergic reactions like seasonal allergic rhinitis, allergic dermatitis, food allergy, drug allergy and insect bite. The histamine released from the mast cells combine with H_1-receptors and mediate allergic symptoms. Therefore, H_1-receptor blockers are used in allergic reactions. The following H_1-blockers (Antihistaminic agents) are available for clinical uses.

1. **Astemizole (Acemiz, Alestol, Astelong, Histalong, Minastem, Perione, Stemiz) :**

   Oral : 10 mg tablets; 5 mg dispersible tablets; 1 mg/mL suspension.

   Dose : Children below 2 years not recommended :

   2-6 years, astemizole suspension 1 mL/5 kg body weight once in a day.

   6-12 years, 5-10 mg once in a day.

   Adult 10 mg once in a day.

2. **Azatadine maleate (Zadine) :**

   Oral : 1 mg tablets.

   Dose : 1-6 years, 1/4 tab twice in a day.

   6-12 years, 1/2 tab twice in a day.

   Adult 1 tab twice in a day.

3. **Brompheniramine maleate (Dimotane) :**

   Oral : 4, 12 mg tablets; Elixir 2 mg/5 mL.

   Dose : 1-3 years, 0.4-1 mg/day in 4 divided doses.

   3-6 years, 2 mg 3-4 times daily.

   6-12 years, 2-4 mg 3-4 times daily.

   Adult, 4-8 mg 3-4 times daily.

4. **Buclizine hydrochloride (Longifene) :**

   Oral : 25 mg tablets; 6 mg/mL syrup.

   Dose : 25-50 mg tablet 30 minutes before dinner for lack of appetite.

5. **Carbinoxamine maleate (Clistin) :**

   Oral : 4 mg tablets.

   Dose : 4-8 mg.

6. **Cetirizine dihydrochloride (Alerid, Allercet, Allerzine, Alzine, Cetrine, Cetzine, Rhizin, Zetop, Zyncet) :**

   Oral : 5, 10 mg tablets; 5 mg/mL syrup.

Dose : Children below 2 years not recommended.

2-6 years, 2.5-5 mg daily.

6-12 years, 5-10 mg daily.

Adult 10 mg daily.

7. **Clemastine fumarate (Tavegyl) :**

Oral : 1 mg tablet; 0.5 mg/5 mL syrup.

Child under 1 year, not recommended.

1-3 years, 250-500 micrograms twice daily.

3-6 years, 500 micrograms twice daily.

6-12 years, 0.5-1 mg twice daily.

Adult 1 mg twice daily.

8. **Cyclizine hydrochloride (Marezine) cyclizine lactate (valoid):**

Oral : 50 mg tablets.

Parenteral : 50 mg/mL for injection.

Dose : 50 mg tab 3 times daily.

50 mg/mL injection by i.m. or i.v. 3 times daily.

9. **Cyproheptadine hydrochloride (Ciplactin, practin) :**

Oral : 4 mg tablets, 2 mg/5 mL syrup.

Dose : 2-6 years, 2 mg 2-3 times daily.

7-14 years, 4 mg 2-3 times daily.

Adult 4 mg, 3-4 times daily.

10. **Dimethindene maleate (Foristal) :**

Oral : 1 mg tablets.

Dose : 2-6 years, 0.5 mg 1-3 times daily.

6-12 years, 1 mg 1-3 times daily.

Adult 2.5 mg 2 times daily.

11. **Dexchlorpheniramine maleate (Polaramine) :**

Dose : 4 months-1 year, 2.5 ml syrup 2-3 times daily.

1 year-5 years, 5 ml 2-3 times daily.

6 years-14 years, 5-7.5 ml 2-3 times daily.

Adults 25 mg 2-3 times daily.

12. **Dimenhydrinate (Dramamine, Gravol) :**

Oral : 50 mg tablets; 15.625 mg/5 mL liquid.

Parenteral : 50 mg/mL for i.m. or i.v. injection.

Dose : 1-6 years 12.5-25 mg, 3-4 times daily.

6-12 years 25-50 mg 3-4 times daily.

Adult 50-100 mg 3-4 times daily.

13. **Diphenhydramine hydrochloride (Benadryl) :**

Oral : 25, 50 mg capsules; 12.5 mg/5 mL syrup.

Dose : 6-12 years, 12.5-25 mg 3-4 times daily.

Adults 25 mg 3-4 times daily.

14. **Embramine hydrochloride (Mebryl) (Mebrophenhydramine) :**

Oral : 25 mg tablets.

Dose : Adults 25-50 mg/day.

15. **Hydroxyzine hydrochloride (Atarax) :**

Oral : 10, 25 mg tablets, 10 mg/5 mL syrup.

Parenteral : 25 mg/mL.

16. **Loratadine (Lorfast) :**

Oral : 10 mg tablets; 5 mg/mL syrup.

Dose : 6-12 years 5 mg once daily.

Adult 10 mg once daily.

17. **Mebhydroline naphadisylate (Incidal) :**

Oral : 50 mg tablets.

Dose : Childre upto 2 years 50 mg/day.

2-5 years 50-150 mg/day.

5-10 years 100-200 mg/day.

Adult and children above 12 years 100-300 mg/day

18. **Meclizine hydrochloride (Diligan) :**

Oral : 12.5 mg tablets.

Dose : Adults 6.26-12.5 mg 3 times daily.

19. **Methdilazine hydrochloride (Dilosyn) :**

Oral : 8 mg tablets; 4 mg/5 mL syrup.

Dose : Children 4 mg 2 times daily.

Adults 8 mg 2 times daily.

20. **Pheniramine maleate (Avil) :**

Oral : 22.5, 45 mg tablets; 15 mg/5 mL syrup.

Parenteral : 22.75 mg/mL.

Dose : 4 months-1 year, 2.5 ml syrup 2-3 times daily.

1 year-5 years, 5 ml 2-3 times daily.

6 years-14 years, 5-7.5 ml 2-3 times daily.

Adults 25 mg 2-3 times daily.

Parenteral adult Dose : 1-2 ml 2 times daily by i.m. injection or by slow i.v. injection. Multidose vials not recommended for i.v. use.

21. **Phenindamine tartrate (Thephorin) :**

Oral : 25 mg tablets.

Dose : Child over 10 years 25 mg 1-3 times daily.

Adult 25-50 mg 1-3 times daily.

22. **Promethazine hydrochloride (Phenergan) :**

Oral : 10, 25 mg tablets; 5 mg/5 mL elixir.

Parenteral : 25 mg/2 mL injection.

Dose : By mouth, child 1-2 years, 5-15 mg 2 times daily.

5-10 years 10-25 mg 2 times daily.

Adult 25 mg 2 times daily.

Parenteral : Child dose (5-10 years) 6.25-12.5 mg by deep intramuscular injection.

Adult Dose : 25-50 mg by i.m. injection.

Slow intravenous injections given in emergencies.

2.5 mg/mL solution in water for injection.

Max. dose given is 25-50 mg (10-50 mL).

23. **Pyrilamine maleate (Frinoz) :**

Nasal drops : 0.02% w/v.

Dose : 2 drops in each nostril 4-6 times a day.

24. **Terfenadine (Tedin, Terdane, Terf, Terfax, Terfed, Tofrin, Trexyl) :**

Oral : 60, 120 mg tablets; 30 mg/5 mL suspension.

Dose : Children under 3 years not recommended.

3-6 years 15 mg 2 times daily.

7-12 years 30 mg 2 times daily.

Adults 60 mg 2 times daily.

120 mg once in a day.

25. **Trimeprazine tartrate (Vallergan) :**
    Oral : 10 mg tablets.
    7.5, 30 mg/5 mL syrup.
    Dose : 2-6 years 2.5-5 mg 3-4 times daily.
    Adults 10 mg 2-3 times daily.
    Elderly 10 mg 1-2 times daily.
26. **Tripelennamine hydrochloride (Pelemine, PBZ) :**
    Oral : 25, 50 mg tablets.
    100 mg sustained release tablets.
    Tripelennamine citrate 37.5 mg/5 mL elixir.
    Dose : 25-50 mg 3 times daily.
27. **Triprolidine hydrochloride (Actidil, Actifed) :**
    Oral : 10 mg tablets.
    Adults 10 mg early evening/day.
    Triprolidine hydrochloride 0.625 mg/5 mL.
    Paediatric suspension :
    2-5 years, 5 ml 3 times daily
    6-12 years 10 ml 3 times daily.

Pharmacist's advise to patients regarding antihistaminics

1. Antihistaminics produce sedation. Therefore, patient should be advised that the drug may affect performance of skilled work (e.g. driving, operation of machines etc.).
2. Antihistaminics should not be given to ladies during pregnancy and lactation period.
3. Antihistaminics are contraindicated in porphyria.

Things to remember about antimuscarinic antispasmodics

Spasmogenic effect due to hypermotility of gastrointestinal tract is mediated partly through the muscarinic receptor activation. Therefore, antimuscarinic agents which are poorly absorbed from gastrointestinal tract are used as antispasmodic agents. The following antispasmodic agents (Antimuscarinic) are available for clinical uses.

1. **Dicyclomine hydrochloride (Merbentyl, spasmo-proxyvon) :**
   Oral : 10, 20 mg tablets; 10 mg/5 mL syrup.

Parenteral : 20 mg/2 mL injection by i.m.

Dose : Not given to infants under 6 months.

6-24 months, 5-10 mg 3-4 times daily 15 minutes before feeds.

2-12 years 10 mg 3 times daily.

Adults 10-20 mg 3 times daily.

2. **Hyoscine butylbromide (Buscopan) :**

   Oral : 10 mg tablets.

   Parenteral : 20 mg/mL injection by i.m. or i.v.

   Dose : 6-12 years 10 mg 3 times daily.

   Adults 20 mg 4 times daily.

3. **Oxyphenonium bromide (Antrenyl) :**

   Oral : 5, 10 mg tablets.

   Dose : 6-12 years 2.5 mg 1-3 times daily.

   Adults 5-10 mg 3-4 times daily.

4. **Propantheline bromide (Pro-banthine) :**

   Oral : 15 mg tablets.

   Dose : Adults 15 mg 3 times daily at least 1 hour before meals.

Pharmacists should advise the patients regarding antimuscarinics

1. Antimuscarinic agents produce visual disturbances like blurring of vision, difficulty with near vision and photophobia.
2. Dryness of mouth.
3. Tachycardia (increase in pulse rate).
4. Retention of urine.

Antimuscarinics are contraindicated in glaucoma, abnormal emptying of bladder, arrhythmias, gastric ulcer, and myasthenia gravis.

EXPERIMENT 13

Identification of unknown sample of drug using guinea pig ileum

AIM

To find out the effect and mechanism of action of the given sample of drug using guinea pig ileum.

PRINCIPLE

Guinea pig ileum is a smooth muscle. Histamine acts on H_1-receptors and produces contraction effect. H_1-blockers antagonise this effect of histamine. Acetylcholine acts on muscarinic receptors and produces contraction effect. Muscarinic blockers antagonise this effect of acetylcholine. Barium chloride produces spasmogenic effect through non-receptor mechanism of action. This action of barium chloride is antagonised by papaverine hydrochloride. Therefore, guinea pig ileum can be used for the identification of H_1-agonists, H_1-antagonists, muscarinic agonists, muscarinic antagonists, non-specific spasmogenic agents and non-specific spasmolytic agents.

REQUIREMENTS

Same as the requirement of Experiment 12.

PROCEDURE

1. Follow steps 1 to 16 of Experiment No. 12.
2. Administer a dose of histamine which produces 50% of the maximal response (EC_{50} dose) and record the response for 30 seconds. Give washings for recovery.
3. Administer a dose of acetylcholine which produces 50% of the maximal response (EC_{50} dose) and record the response for 30 seconds. Give washings for recovery.
4. Administer a dose of barium chloride which produces 50% of the maximal response (EC_{50} dose) and record the response for 30 seconds. Give washings for recovery.
5. Add 0.1 ml of the given test sample solution into the inner organ bath and record the response for 30 seconds. If the test sample

produces contraction of the guinea pig ileum, it indicates that the given sample is either an agonist or a non-specific spasmogenic agent.

6. **Identification of H_1-agonist :** Add 0.1 ml of chlorpheniramine into the inner organ bath and allow it to act for 2 minutes. Then add 0.1 ml of the given test sample into the inner organ bath and record the response for 30 seconds. Failure of the test sample to produce a contraction effect in the presence of H_1-blocker indicates that the given sample is a H_1-receptor agonist.

   If the test sample shows contraction effect in the presence of a H_1-blocker it indicates that the given sample is not a H_1-receptor agonist.

7. **Identification of muscarinic agonist :** Add 0.1 ml of atropine sulphate solution into the inner organ bath and allow it to act for 2 minutes. Then add 0.1 ml of the given test sample into the inner organ bath and record the response for 30 seconds. Failure of the test sample to produce contraction effect in the presence of a muscarinic blocker confirms that the given sample is a muscarinic receptor agonist. If the test sample shows contraction effect in the presence of a muscarinic blocker it indicates that the given sample is not a muscarinic agonist.

8. **Identification of non-specific spasmogenic agent :** Add 0.1 ml of papaverine hydrochloride solution into the inner organ bath and allow it to act for 2 minutes. Then add 0.1 ml of the test sample and record the response for 30 seconds. Failure of the test sample to produce contraction effect in the presence of a non-specific spasmolytic agent indicates that the given sample is a non-specific spasmogenic agent.

9. **Identification of an antagonist :** Add 0.1 ml of the test sample into the inner organ bath and observe. If the test sample fails to produce any response it indicates that it may be an antagonist or Tyrode solution or distilled water.

   (a) *Identification of a H_1-receptor blocker :* Add 0.1 ml of the test sample into the inner organ bath and allow it to act for 2 minutes. Then record the effect of EC_{50} dose of histamine in the presence of test sample. If the effect of EC_{50} dose of histamine is reduced it confirms that the given test solution contains a H_1-receptor blocker.

   (b) *Identification of muscarinic blocker :* Add 0.1 ml of the test sample into the inner organ bath and allow it to act for 2 minutes. Then record the effect of EC_{50} dose of acetylcholine in the presence of test sample. If the effect of EC_{50} dose of acetylcholine is reduced it confirms that the given test solution is a muscarinic blocker.

(c) *Identification of non-specific spasmolytic agent* : Add 0.1 ml of the test sample into the inner organ bath and allow it to act for 2 minutes, then record the effect of EC_{50} dose of barium chloride in the presence of the test sample. If the effect of EC_{50} dose of barium chloride is reduced, it indicates that the given sample is a non-specific spasmolytic agent.

N.B. : If test solution does not modify the responses of standard drugs (histamine, acetylcholine, barium chloride) it indicates that the given test solution does not contain any drug.

EXPERIMENT 14

Effect of spasmogens and relaxants on rabbit intestine

AIM

To study the effects of acetylcholine, physostigmine, and adrenaline on rabbit intestine.

PRINCIPLE

Rabbit intestine is a smooth muscle which shows regular pendular movement (i.e. continuous contraction and relaxation). Therefore, to study the effect of drugs on intestinal movement rabbit intestine is an ideal preparation. Rabbit intestine is supplied by autonomic nervous system. Rabbit intestine contains muscarinic receptors and adrenergic receptors. Muscarinic receptor agonist like acetylcholine produces contraction of rabbit intestine and physostigmine increases the spasm and pendular movements. The above muscarinic actions and effects can be blocked by muscarinic blockers.

Adrenaline acts on alpha and beta receptors and exhibits inhibitory effect on pendular movements. The actions of adrenaline is blocked by adrenoceptor blockers like alpha receptor blockers and beta receptor blockers.

EQUIPMENTS REQUIRED

INCO kymograph, student thermostatic organ bath, aeration tube, aeration tube holder, frontal writing lever, lever holder, screw clip, haemostatic forceps, Mariotte bottle, rubber tubes, tuberculine syringe, 26 No. needle, suturing needle, scissor, forceps, carbogen gas cylinder with regulator.

Animal required

Rabbit.

Physiological solution required

Tyrode solution.

Drug solution required

1. Acetylcholine chloride 20 microgram/mL.

2. Physostigmine sulphate 10 microgram/mL.
3. Atropine sulphate 4 microgram/mL.
4. Adrenaline hydrogen tartrate 20 microgram/mL.
5. Propranolol hydrochloride 100 microgram/mL.

PROCEDURE

1. Fast a rabbit for 12 hour period.
2. Set up the assembly for rabbit intestine experiment.
3. Balance a frontal writing lever using plasticine and apply a tension of 500 mg.
4. Fill the outer jacket of student organ bath with water.
5. Set the thermostat of the student organ bath at 37°C and put the switch on.
6. Fill the mariotte bottle with Tyrode solution and control the flow of Tyrode solution to the inner organ bath using haemostatic forceps.
7. When the temperature of the Tyrode solution reaches 37°C, kill a rabbit by giving a blow on its head and cutting the carotid artery.
8. Open the abdominal region and identify the intestine.
9. Remove a length of intestine and place it in a petri dish containing Tyrodes solution at 37°C and trim away the mesentery.
10. Cut a piece of intestine (approximately 3-4 cm) and using surgical suturing needle tie a thread at each end, taking care to see that the lumen of the intestine remained open.
11. Tie one end of the thread to the hook of the aeration tube and the other to a frontal writing lever.
12. Stabilize the tissue for 30 minutes period.
13. Aerate the rabbit intestine in the inner organ bath with a mixture of oxygen (95 per cent) and carbon dioxide (5 per cent) (carbogen).
15. Record the normal pendular movement of the rabbit intestine on the drum for 30 seconds. At the end of 30 seconds add 0.1 ml of acetylcholine into the inner organ bath and record the spasmogenic effect of the drug for 30 seconds. After recording the response for 30 seconds switch off the kymograph. Immediately open the outlet of the inner organ bath and remove the

Tyrode's solution present in the inner organ bath. Again fill the inner organ bath with fresh Tyrode's solution and keep it for 60 seconds. Repeat the washing procedure 3-4 times or till the writing point of frontal lever comes to the normal pendular movement base line.

16. Then record the response of 0.1 ml physostigmine solution. Give 3-4 washings for recovery.

17. Record the response of 0.1 ml adrenaline solution. Give 3-4 washings for recovery.

18. Add 0.1 ml of atropine sulphate solution into the inner organ bath, allow it to act for 60 seconds then record the response of acetylcholine in the presence of atropine sulphate. Give-3-4 washings for recovery.

19. Add 0.1 ml of atropine sulphate solution into the inner organ bath, allow it to act for 60 seconds then record the response of physostigmine solution in the presence of atropine sulphate. Give 3-4 washings for recovery.

20. Add 0.1 ml of propranolol solution into the inner organ bath, allow it to act for 60 seconds then record the response of adrenaline solution in the presence of propranolol. Give 3-4 washings for recovery.

OBSERVATION AND CONCLUSION

Acetylcholine produced contraction of the rabbit intestine. Atropine sulphate is a muscarinic receptor blocker, therefore it reduced the spasmogenic effect caused by acetylcholine.

Physostigmine also produced mild spasmogenic effect and increased the peristallic movement of the intestine. Atropine sulphate blocked the effect of physostigmine.

Things to remember

1. Antimuscarinic agents which are poorly absorbed from gastrointestinal tract are used as antispasmodic agents.

2. Anticholine esterase agents like neostigmine bromide which does not cross the blood brain barrier can be used in atonic constipation. The preparation available is Neostigmine bromide (Tilstigmin).

Oral : 15 mg tablets.

Dose : 15 mg four times daily.

Physostigmine is not preferred for atonic constipation because it crosses blood brain barrier and produces CNS side effects.

Adrenaline produced relaxation of rabbit intestine. This effect is partly blocked by propranolol. The above observation indicates that adrenaline acts both on alpha and beta receptors.

CHAPTER 6
Drugs Acting on Eye

EXPERIMENT 15
Effect of mydriatics and miotics on rabbit eye

AIM

1. To study the effect of mydriatics (Antimuscarinics) like atropine sulphate, cyclopentolate hydrochloride homatropine hydrobromide and tropicamide on rabbit eye.

2. To study the effect of mydriatics (alpha-1 receptor agonists) like adrenaline hydrochloride, dipivefrine hydrochloride and phenylephrine hydrochloride.

3. To study the effects of miotics (muscarinic agonists) like carbachol and pilocarpine nitrate on rabbit eye.

4. To study the effect of miotic (Anticholinesterase agent) like physostigmine sulphate on rabbit eye.

5. To measure the intraocular pressure of the rabbit eye before and after the administration of miotic.

PRINCIPLE

Antimuscarinics cause reversible paralysis of constrictor pupillae (circular muscle of iris) and ciliary muscle which leads to mydriasis, cycloplegia and increased intraocular pressure. Alpha-1 receptor agonists cause contraction of dilator pupillae (radial muscle of iris) and produce mydriasis. Alpha-1 receptor agonists do not increase intraocular pressure.

Muscarinic agonists cause contraction of constrictor pupillae (the circular muscle of iris) and ciliary muscle and reduction of intraocular pressure.

Anticholinesterase agents inhibit cholineesterase enzyme and increase the concentration of acetylcholine and thus exhibit muscarinic activity on the eye.

EQUIPMENTS REQUIRED

Schioetz-Tonometer, Pentorch, dropper.

Animal required

Rabbits.

Drug solutions required

A. **Mydriatics (Antimuscarinics) :**
   Atropine sulphate 1% w/v.
   Cyclopentolate hydrochloride 1% w/v.
   Homatropine hydrobromide 1% w/v.
   Tropicamide 0.5% w/v.

B. **Mydriatics (Alpha-1 receptor agonist) :**
   Adrenaline hydrochloride 1% w/v.
   Dipivefrine hydrochloride 0.1% w/v.
   Phenylephrine hydrochloride 5% w/v.

C. **Miotics (Muscarinic receptor agonist) :**
   Carbachol 3% w/v.
   Pilocarpine nitrate 1% w/v.

D. **Miotic (Anticholine esterase agent) :**
   Physostigmine sulphate 0.25% w/v.

E. **Local anaesthetic required for measuring intraocular pressure :**
   Lignocaine hydrochloride 4% w/v.

   Depending upon the availability, teachers can select any one of the drugs mentioned in each category.

PROCEDURE

1. Select six healthy albino rabbits weighing between 1.5 to 2 kg body weight and do the marking for identification of each rabbit.

2. Observe the size of the pupil of each rabbit using a pentorch.

3. Instil the eye drops of the following drugs as given below :

Name of the drug	Dose	Rabbit No.
Cyclopentolate hydrochloride	2-3 drops	1
Phenylephrine hydrochloride	2-3 drops	2
Pilocarpine nitrate	2-3 drops	3
Physostigmine sulphate	2-3 drops	4

Normal saline	2-3 drops	5
Lignocaine hydrochloride	2-3 drops ⎫	
After 5 minutes	⎬	6
Pilocarpine nitrate	2-3 drops ⎭	

4. Observe the size of the pupil of each rabbit at 30 minutes interval for a period of 2 hours (Rabbit No. 1-4).
5. Adjust the Schioetz-Tonometer pointer on zero position.
6. Place the tonometer in a vertical position on the center of the cornea (Rabbit No. 5-6).
7. Read the position of the pointer and calculate the tension in mm Hg (Intraocular pressure) by the table.

OBSERVATION AND CONCLUSION

Cyclopentolate hydrochloride produced dilatation of the pupil due to antimuscarinic activity. Phenylephrine hydrochloride also produced dilatation of the pupil because of alpha-1 receptor stimulation.

Pilocarpine nitrate produced miosis of the pupil and reduced intraocular pressure due to muscarinic receptor activation.

Physostigmine sulphate produced effect similar to pilocarpine.

Things to remember

Mydriatics and Miotics are clinically used for diagnosis and therapy of ocular disorders. The following drugs are available for diagnosis and clinical uses.

A. **Mydriatics (Antimuscarinics) :**

1. Cyclopentolate hydrochloride 1% eye drops (cyclogic eye drops).

2. Tropicamide 1% w/v (Tropisyn eye drops).

   Antimuscarinic mydriatics are used for producing mydriasis and cycloplegia in diagnostic procedures. (For accurate measurement of refractive error, examination of retina.) Tropicamide is used whenever short action is required. Atropine is used for the treatment of iridocyclitis.

B. **Mydriatic (alpha-1-receptor agonist) :**

   Phenylephrine hydrochloride 5, 10% w/v (Drosyn eye drops).

   Phenylephrine hydrochloride is used as a mydriatic in ophthalmoscopic examination (For funduscopic examination).

It lowers intraocular pressure by increasing aqueous outflow.

C. **Miotic (Muscarinic receptor agonist) :**

Pilocarpine nitrate 1% w/v (Pilocar).

Pilocarpine is used in glaucoma (open angle glaucoma).

Note : In angle closure glaucoma surgery (Iridectomy) is done.

Pharmacist's advise for the patients

Pharmacists should warn the patients, not to drive for 1-2 hours after mydriasis.

Other drugs used in the treatment of glaucoma

Glaucoma occurs due to defect in drainage of aqueous humor and this results in a rise of intraocular pressure. The normal intraocular pressure is between 15-25 mm Hg. Glaucoma if not corrected leads to blindness.

Beta-receptors blocking agents are also used in glaucoma. High concentration of cyclic adenosine monophosphate (cAMP) increases the formation of aqueous humor and precipitates glaucoma. Beta-receptor blockers lower the formation of aqueous humor and reduces intraocular pressure. Therefore, beta-receptor blockers are used in glaucoma. The following beta-receptor blockers are available for clinical uses.

1. **Betaxolol hydrochloride (Optipress, opteze, iobet) :**

    Tropical : 0.25, 0.5% w/v eye drops.

    Dose : 1-2 drops twice in a day.

2. **Timolol maleate (Glaucare, Glucotim, Iotim) :**

    Tropical : 0.25, 0.5% w/v eye drops.

    Dose : 1 drop twice in a day.

CHAPTER 7
Local Anaesthetics

EXPERIMENT 16

Bioevaluation technique for local anaesthetic activity

AIM

(a) To study the local anaesthetic activity of Lignocaine hydrochloride on rabbit cornea (surface anaesthesia method).

(b) To study the local anaesthetic activity of Lignocaine hydrochloride or procaine hydrochloride using infiltration technique in guinea pigs. (Infiltration anaesthesia method).

(c) To study the local anaesthetic activity of Lignocaine hydrochloride using nerve block technique in frogs.

(Nerve block anaesthesia method)

PRINCIPLE

Local anaesthesia is the condition that results when sensory input from a local area to the central nervous system is blocked. Local anaesthetics are drugs which reversibly block conduction of impulses along nerve axons and excitable membrane.

(A) EVALUATION OF LOCAL ANAESTHETIC ACTIVITY OF LIGNOCAINE HYDROCHLORIDE ON RABBIT CORNEA.

EQUIPMENT REQUIRED

Stop watch, Rabbit cages to keep rabbits in place, dropper, camel hair.

Animal required : Albino rabbits.

Drug solution required

Lignocaine hydrochloride 0.1%, 0.2%, 0.4%, 0.5%, 1% and 2%.

PROCEDURE

1. Select six healthy albino rabbits weighing about 1.5 to 2 kg body weight.

2. Trim their eye lashes one day before the experiment.

3. Keep each rabbit separately in a rabbit cage and number the cage.

4. Instil the lowest concentration of lignocaine hydrochloride solution on the corneal surface of the rabbit, so that the space between eyelids contained a clearly visible film of the solution. Note the time of administration of drug solution.

5. Stimulate the cornea by touching it with a camel hair a minute after instillation.

6. Stimulate the cornea at 60 seconds interval for a period of 30 minutes.

7. Count the number of times the animal fails to respond to a corneal stimuli during 30 minutes period.

8. Find out the onset of action, duration of action and degree of anaesthesia.

OBSERVATION AND CONCLUSION

Local application of lignocaine hydrochloride solution produced loss of sensation at the site of application. The above observation indicates that lignocaine hydrochloride is a surface anaesthetic agent.

(B) EVALUATION OF LOCAL ANAESTHETIC ACTIVITY OF LIGNOCAINE HYDROCHLORIDE USING INFILTRATION TECHNIQUE IN GUINEA PIGS

EQUIPMENTS REQUIRED

Stop watch, cages for keeping guinea pigs, 26 No. needle, electric stimulator, hair clipper.

Animal required

Guinea pigs.

Other materials required

Hair remover (Anne French), marking pens.

Drugs required

1. Lignocaine hydrochloride 20 mg/mL or Procaine hydrochloride 20 mg/mL.

2. Normal saline (0.9% NaCl).

PROCEDURE

1. Select six guinea pigs weighing about 200-300 g body weight.

2. Remove the hair on the backs of these animals by using hair clipper, one day before the experiment. Apply Anne French hair remover on the shaved backs of these animals. Allow the Anne French cream to make contact with the skin for 5 minutes. Using a damp surgical cotton/towel and warm water wash off the Anne French cream from the backs of these animals.

3. Inject 3 animals with 0.25 mL normal saline intradermally using 26 No. needle.

4. Inject the other 3 animals with 0.25 ml of 0.1% Lignocaine hydrochloride solution intradermally. Note the time of injection.

5. Mark the injected area with marker ink.

6. Five minutes after the injection, stimulate the injected area through a bipolar electrode (0.25 mA current for 2-3 seconds) connected to a stimulator.

   If stimulator is not available, stimulate the injected area by pricking with a 27 No. needle. Give 6 stimulation at 5 seconds interval. Repeat the procedure at 5 minutes interval.

7. Continue the stimulation procedure for 30 minutes.

8. Note the time when the tissue is insensitive to stimuli (on set of action).

9. Note the time when the tissue is sensitive to stimuli (Duration of action).

10. Find out the percentage degree of anaesthesia.

   e.g. $\dfrac{\text{Number of insensitive response}}{\text{Total number of stimuli}} = \dfrac{36}{36}$ indicates

   100% anaesthesia

   $\dfrac{\text{Number of insensitive response (18)}}{\text{Total number of stimuli (36)}}$ indicates

   50% anaesthesia.

OBSERVATION AND CONCLUSION

Intradermal injection of Lignocaine hydrochloride produced loss of sensation around the area of injection site. The observation indicates that lignocaine hydrochloride produces infiltration anaesthesia. Infiltration anaesthesia is used for minor operation.

(C) EVALUATION OF LOCAL ANAESTHETIC ACTIVITY OF LIGNOCAINE HYDROCHLORIDE USING NERVE BLOCK TECHNIQUE IN FROGS

PRINCIPLE

Hydrochloric acid produces irritant effect on the frog skin. When frog's foot is dipped in N/10 hydrochloric acid it reflexly withdraws it. Substances which block the generation and conduction of impulse in nerve fibres should, therefore block this reflex effect when applied to the sciatic nerve.

EQUIPMENTS REQUIRED

Spotwatch, T-rod, L-stand, surgical instruments, 250 ml beakers.

Animal required

Frogs.

Chemicals and drug solution required

N/10 hydrochloric acid, normal saline (0.9% NaCl), lignocaine hydrochloride.

PROCEDURE

1. Hold a frog in the left hand and make a cut at the occipito-atlantic junction between the brain and spinal cord using a sharp scalpel.
2. Using a pithing needle decerebrate the frog.
3. Make a lateral cut high up across the abdomen.
4. Remove all the abdominal organs so that a sac is formed of abdominal walls.
5. Tie the fore limbs of the frog to a T-rod in such a way that its hind legs hang free.
6. Immerse the right hind leg of the frog in the beaker containing N/10 hydrochloric acid and observe the brisk withdrawal. Wash the leg immediately with tap water.

7. Immerse the left hind leg of the frog in a beaker containing normal saline and observe the absence of leg withdrawal.

8. Place the lignocaine hydrochloride solution (0.5% 10 ml) in the abdominal sac and note the time.

9. Test the withdrawal reflex once a minute, using N/10 hydrochloric acid, remembering always to wash off the acid afterwards.

10. Observe the time required for the reflex withdrawal of legs.

OBSERVATION AND CONCLUSION

When lignocaine hydrochloride is applied in close proximity to the sciatic nerve the hind legs are anaesthetized. This observation indicates that lignocaine hydrochloride injection can be used for regional nerve block anaesthesia.

Things to remember

The following local anasthetis are available for clinical uses.

1. **Benzocaine :**

   Tropical

   1% w/v.

   Chloromycetin ear drops contain chloromycetin 5% w/v and benzocaine 1% w/v. Benzocaine is used as a surface anaesthetic agent for the relief of pain and irritation.

2. **Bupivacaine (Anawin injection) :**

   Parenteral

   5 mg/mL.

   Dose : Local infiltration 0.25% (upto 60 ml).

   Peripheral nerve block 0.25% (upto 60 ml)

   0.5% (upto 30 ml)

   Epidural block :

   Surgery Lumbar 0.5% (20 ml)

   Labour Lumbar 0.25-0.5% (upto 12 ml)

   Bupivacaine HCl 5 mg/ml ⎫
           +   ⎬ 2-4 ml for spinal anaesthesia
   Glucose 80 mg/mL ⎭

3. **Dibucaine (otogesic) :**

   Tropical : 1.1% ear drops along with other drugs.

4. **Lignocaine hydrochloride (xylocaine, lidocaine gescicam, lox):**

   Tropical : 2-4% is used for surface anaesthesia-max dose 200 mg.

   Dental spray : 10-50 mg.

   Parenteral : Infiltration 4.5 mg/kg

   Nerve block 1% solution (upto 50 mL)

   Epidural and caudal block 1% (upto 50 ml)

5. **Procaine hydrochloride :**

   Parenteral : 0.5% (upto 200 ml)

   Not widely used.

Pharmacist should advise the surgeon regarding the following properties of local anaesthetics

1. Local anaesthetics should not be injected into inflammed or infected tissues, nor should be applied to traumatised urethra because toxicity will be produced.

2. Adrenaline containing local anaesthetics should not be injected into tissues supplied by end arteries e.g. fingers, toes, ears, nose, penis, because gangrene may develop.

CHAPTER 8
Drugs Acting on Central Nervous System

EXPERIMENT NO. 17

Effect of strychnine in frog

AIM

To study the central nervous system stimulant and convulsant effect of strychnine hydrochloride in frog.

PRINCIPLE

Strychnine is a powerful central nervous system stimulant and convulsant. The main site of action of strychnine is spinal cord. Glycine is an inhibitory neurotransmitter present in the spinal cord.Strychnine antagonises the action of glycine and produces convulsion.

APPARATUS REQUIRED : 26 No. needle, plastic cages.

Animal required : Frog.

Drug solutions required

1. Normal saline (sodium chloride 0.9% w/v).
2. Strychnine hydrochloride 4 mg/mL.

PROCEDURE

1. Weigh six frogs and divide them into two groups each comprising of three frogs and keep them in a plastic cage.
2. Administer normal saline (1 ml/kg body weight) to group I by subcutaneous injection.
3. Administer strychnine hydrochloride (4 mg/kg body weight) subcutaneously to group II and note the time of administration of strychnine hydrochloride.
4. Observe the onset, severity and duration of hyperreflex activity and convulsion produced in each frog.

Observations may be recorded as given below :

Group I (control) Normal saline 1 mL/kg SC

S.No.	Body weight of frog g	Hyper reflex activity	Observation Convulsion	Mortality
1.	200	Nil	Nil	Nil
2.	160	Nil	Nil	Nil
3.	190	Nil	Nil	Nil

Group II (Drug treated) strychnine hydrochloride 4 mg/kg SC

S.No.	Body weight of frog g	Hyper reflex activity	Observation Convulsion	Mortality
1.	190			
2.	200			
3.	160			

OBSERVATION AND CONCLUSION

Strychnine hydrochloride produced hyper reflex activity followed by convulsion. The above observations indicate that strychnine is a stimulant and convulsant.

Note : Strychnine is not clinically used.

EXPERIMENT 18

Effect of convulsants and anticonvulsants in mice

AIMS

A. To measure the property of diazepam or sodium valproate to suppress chemoshock (convulsion induced by pentylenetetrazole or picrotoxin) in mice.

PRINCIPLE

Central nervous system stimulants at higher doses produce convulsion. Pentylenetetrazole closes the GABA-linked chloride channels in the brain. Therefore, it produces clonic convulsion. Diazepam and sodium valproate open the GABA linked chloride channels and produce hyperpolarization. Therefore, they prevent the convulsion induced by pentylene tetrazole or picrotoxin. Compounds which prevent chemoshock are found to be useful in treating absence - seizure (petitmal epilepsy).

EQUIPMENTS AND OTHER MATERIALS REQUIRED

Stop watch, plastic mice cages, disposable syringes 26 No. needle.

Animal

Mice.

Drug solution required

Diazepam 0.5 mg/mL

Sodium valproate 30 mg/mL

Pentylene tetrazole 8 mg/mL

Picrotoxin 0.8 mg/mL

PROCEDURE

1. Select 15 albino mice having body weight between 20-25 g.
2. Divide the mice into three groups of five animals.
3. Weigh the mouse in each group, do the marking and keep them in mice cages.
4. Administer the drug solutions as shown below :

Group I : Pentylene tetrazole 80 mg/kg i.p. or Picrotoxin 4 mg/kg i.p.

Group II : Inject diazepam 5 mg/kg i.p. After 30 minutes inject pentylenetetrazole 80 mg/kg i.p. or Picrotoxin 4 mg/kg i.p.

Group III : Administer Sodium valproate 300 mg/kg p.o. after 90 minutes inject pentylene tetrazole 80 mg/kg i.p. or Picrotoxin 4 mg/kg i.p.

5. Record the observations as shown below :

Group I : Pentylenetetrazole 80 mg/kg i.p.

S. No.	Markings	Body weight in g	Dose in mg	ml	Time of injection	Observations	
						Convulsion	Mortality
1.	Head						
2.	Back						
3.	Tail						
4.	Head & Back						
5.	Head & Tail						

Observe the onset and duration of convulsion and their type (tonic or clonic).

6. Record the observations for group II and group III.

OBSERVATION AND CONCLUSION

1. The group which received pentylene-tetrazole showed clonic convulsions.

2. Diazepam pretreatment protected the mice against pentylene-tetrazole induced convulsion.

3. Sodium valproate pretreatment protected the mice against pentylenetetrazole induced convulsion.

4. Diazepam and sodium valproate are used in convulsive disorders.

Things to remember

1. Diazepam is given intravenously in the treatment of status epilepsy.

   Dose : Children : 200-300 micrograms/kg body weight.

   Adults : 10-20 mg at a rate of 2.5 mg/30 seconds.

2. The following drugs are used in the treatment of petitmal epilepsy.

(a) **Clonazepam (Lonazep, Rivotril) :**

Oral : 0.5, 2 mg tablets.

Dose : Infants and children 0.01-0.02 mg/kg/day in 3-4 divided doses.

(b) **Sodium valproate (Epilex) :**

Oral : 200 mg/5 mL solution.

Dose : Children under 20 kg : 20 mg/kg/day in divided doses. Children above 20 kg 50 mg/kg/day in divided doses.

To measure the property of diphenylhydantoin sodium (Dilantin sodium) to suppress Maximal Electroshock Seizures (MES) in mice.

PRINCIPLE

MES test is used to find out drugs that prevent spread of seizures. Maximal Electroshock produces convulsive symptoms similar to grandmal epilepsy. Therefore, drugs which prevent MES are usually found to be useful in the treatment of grandmal epilepsy.

EQUIPMENTS AND OTHER MATERIALS REQUIRED

Electroshock apparatus (Electroconvulsometer) corneal electrodes or ear electrodes, stop watch, mice cages, disposable syringes and 26 No. needle.

Animal

Mice.

Drug solutions required

1. Normal saline (0.9% sodium chloride).
2. Dilantin sodium 4 mg/mL.
3. Phenobarbitone sodium 3 mg/mL.

PROCEDURE

1. Select 15 mice having body weight between 20-25 g.
2. Divide the mice into three groups of five animals.

3. Weigh the mouse in each group, do the marking and keep them in mice cages.

4. Administer the drug solution as shown below :

   Group I : Normal saline 1 ml/kg i.p.

   Group II : Dilantin sodium 40 mg/kg i.p.

   Group III : Phenobarbitone sodium 30 mg/kg i.p.

5. Return each group to their respective cages.

6. Set up the electroconvulsometer to deliver a current of 50 mA for 0.2 sec duration either through corneal electrodes or ear electrodes.

7. After 30 minutes, apply MES to each mouse by placing a pair of corneal electrodes directly to the eye balls or by placing a pair of ear electrodes.

8. Immediately after applying MES observe the duration of tonic and clonic convulsion in each mouse. The duration is usually more than 10 seconds. If the duration is less than 10 seconds it indicates that test compound is active.

9. Record the observations as shown below :

   Group I : Normal saline 1 mL/kg i.p.

S. No.	Markings	Body weight in g	Dose	Time of injection	Observations Duration of Convulsion		
					Tonic	Clonic	Mortality
1.	Head						
2.	Back						
3.	Tail						
4.	Head & back						
5.	Head & tail						

MES produces tonic convulsion (characterized by extension of hind limbs) and clonic convulsion (characterized by continuous cycling motion of limbs).

10. Record the observations for group II and group III.

OBSERVATIONS AND CONCLUSIONS

1. The group which received normal saline showed tonic extensor phase and clonic phase convulsion and the duration was more than 10 seconds.

2. The group which received dilantin sodium did not exhibit the extensor phase of convulsion.

3. The group which received phenobarbitone sodium did not exhibit extensor phase of convulsion.

4. Drugs which prevent MES are useful in the treatment of grandmal epilepsy.

Things to remember

Drugs used in the treatment of grand-mal epilepsy act by multiple mechanisms. Dilantin sodium prolong the inactivation of Na^+ channels.

Barbiturates open the chloride channels.

Sodium valproate open the chloride channels also reduce the flow Ca^{++} through T-type Ca^{++} channels.

The following drugs are used as anticonvulsants in the treatment of grand mal epilepsy.

1. **Carbamazepine (Carmaz, Mazetol, Mezapin, Tegretol, Zen-Retard, Zen, Zeptol) :**

   Oral : 100, 200 mg tablets, 400 mg tablets; 100 mg/5 mL suspension.

   Dose : Children upto 1 year 100-200 mg/day 1-2 times daily

   1-5 years 200-400 mg/day 1-2 times daily

   6-10 years 400-600 mg/day 1-2 times daily

   11-15 years 600-1000 mg/day 1-2 times daily

   Adults 800-1200 mg/day 1-2 times daily.

2. **Gabapentin (Neurontin) :**

   Oral : 300, 400 mg capsules.

   Dose : Adults and children above 12 years — 900-1800 mg/day in divided doses. Maximum dose 2400 mg/day in divided doses.

3. **Phenobarbitone (Beetal, Gardenal, Luminal) :**

   Oral : 30, 60 mg tablets.

   Dose : Children : 3 mg/kg/day at bed time. Adults : 30-200 mg/ day in divided doses.

4. **Phenobarbitone sodium injection :**

   200 mg/mL injection

   Dose : For sedation : Children : 1-3 mg/kg i.m. or i.v.

   Adults : 100-200 mg i.m.

For hypnosis :

Adults : 100-320 mg i.m. or i.v.

For acute convulsion :

Children : 4-6 mg/kg/day i.m. or i.v.

Adults : 200-320 mg i.m. or i.v.

For status epilepticus :

Adults : 15-20 mg/kg i.v. over 15-20 minutes.

5. **Phenytoin sodium or Diphenylhydantoin or Dilantin sodium (Dilantin, Eptoin) :**

   Oral : 100 mg capsules; 100 mg/4 mL suspension.

   Dose : Children under 6 years : 25-50 mg 2-4 times daily. Children over 6 years : 100 mg 3-4 times daily. Adults : 100 mg 3-4 times daily.

6. **Primidone (Mysoline) :**

   Oral : 250 mg tablets.

   Dose : Initial 125 mg at bed time.

   Gradually increase every 3 days by 125 mg maximum dose 500 mg/day.

7. **Sodium valproate (Encorate, Epilex, Valparin, Valprol) :**

   Oral : 200, 500 mg tablets; 200 mg/5 mL solution.

   Dose : Children under 20 kgs : 20 mg/kg body wt/day into two doses after meals.

   Children over 20 kgs : 50 mg/kg body wt/day into two doses after meals.

   Adults : Initial dose 600 mg/day in two divided doses. Gradually increase by 200 mg at 3 days interval to maximum of 2600 mg/ day.

Pharmacists should advise the patients regarding the significances of estimating the blood concentration of phenytoin during therapy. Because phenytoin has narrow margin of safety. Estimations of the plasma concentration of other antiepileptics are also essential for optimal therapy.

EXPERIMENT 19

Effect of hypnotics in mice

AIM

To study the sedative and hypnotic effects of benzodiazepines and barbiturates.

PRINCIPLE

Sedative drugs suppress the responsiveness to a constant stimulation. Sedative drugs decrease the spontaneous motor activity.

Hypnotics are drugs which induce sleep resembling natural sleep.

Hypnotics in higher doses (e.g. Pentobarbitone sodium, hexobarbitone sodium) produce anaesthesia.

The benzodiazepines and barbiturates bind to $GABA_A$-receptor. (GABA = gamma amino butyric acid).

Benzodiazepines (e.g. Diazepam, Flurazepam, Nitrazepam etc.) increase the frequency of opening of chloride channel.

Barbiturates increase the duration of opening of chloride channel.

Barbiturates also inhibit excitatory AMPA (DL alpha amino 3-hydroxy 5-methyl isoxazole 4 propionate) glutamate receptors.

Thus bendodiazepines and barbiturates act as central nervous system depressants.

EQUIPMENTS AND OTHER MATERIALS REQUIRED

Actophotometer, stop watch, mouse cages disposable 26 No. needles, disposable syringes.

Animal

Albino mice.

Drug solutions required

1. Normal saline (sodium chloride 0.9% w/v).
2. Phenobarbitone sodium 3 mg/mL.
3. Pentobarbitone sodium 4 mg/mL.

4. Nitrazepam 0.5 mg/mL.

PROCEDURE

1. Select 20 albino mice having body weight between 25-30 g.
2. Fast the mice for 12 hours before the experiment.
3. Divide the mice into four groups of five animals.
4. Weigh the mouse in each group do the marking and keep them in plastic cages.
5. Put each group of mice into a Actophotometer and record their motor activity for 30 minutes.
6. After 30 minutes remove each group of mice from the Actophotometer.
7. Administer the drug solutions as shown below :

   Group I : Normal saline 1 ml/100 g i.p.

   Group II : Phenobarbitone sodium 30 mg/kg i.p.

   Group III : Pentobarbitone sodium 40 mg/kg i.p.

   Group IV : Nitrazepam 5 mg/kg orally.

8. Record the observations as shown below :

   Group I : Control normal saline 1 ml/kg i.p.

S. No.	Markings	Body weight in g	Dose in ml	Time of injection	Motor Activity	Sedation	LRR
1.	Head	25	0.25				
2.	Back	30	0.3				
3.	Tail	50	0.3				
4.	Head and back	25	0.25				
5.	Head & tail	25	0.25				

LRR = Loss of righting reflex.

Make similar table for Group II, III and IV and record the observations.

OBSERVATIONS AND CONCLUSION

1. The group which received normal saline showed spontaneous motor activity and the count was...............

2. The group which received phenobarbitone sodium showed decrease in spontaneous motor activity.

3. The group which received pentobarbitone sodium showed loss of righting reflex.

4. The group which received nitrazepam showed decrease in motor activity.

5. Therefore, barbiturates and benzodiazepines are used as sedatives and hypnotics.

Things to remember

Sedative-hypnotics will induce sleep. Therefore, sedative-hypnotics are used in insomnia. The following drugs are available for clinical uses.

Benzodiazepines

Note : Benzodiazepines have anxiolytic properties. Therefore, they are used as sedative-hypnotics and anxiolytic agents.

1. **Alprazolam (Alprax, Alzolam, Alzomax, Alzopax, Anxit, Anxyl, Nitril Plaxid, Quiet, Restyl, Sozo, Tranisol, Trika, Trizo, Xanti, Zenax, Zenoprax, Zolam, Zolax, Zoldac, Zopic):**

   Oral : 0.25, 0.5, 1 mg tablets.

   Dose : Children not recommended.

   Adults : 0.25-1 mg 2-3 times in a day.

   Elderly : 0.25 mg 2-3 times in a day.

   Alprazolam is mainly used as an anti-anxiety agent.

2. **Chlordiazepoxide hydrochloride (Librium) :**

   Oral : 10 mg tablets.

   Dose : Children 5-10 mg 3 times daily.

   Adults : 20-40 mg 3 times daily.

   Elderly : 10-20 mg 3 timesdaily.

   Use : Anxiolytic.

3. **Diazepam (Anxol, Calmpose, Camrelease, Dizep, Elcion, Lori, Placidox, Valium) :**

   Oral : 5, 10 mg tablets; 2 mg/5 mL suspension.

   10, 15 mg controlled release capsules.

   Parenteral : 5 mg/mL injection i.m. or i.v.

Dose : Children upto 3 years 1-6 mg at bed time.

Children 4-14 years 4-12 mg 2 times daily.

Adults : 2.5-10 mg 2-4 times daily.

Elderly : 2.5-5 mg at bed time as a hypnotic.

Use : Anxiolytic, hypnotic.

4. **Flurazepam (Nindral) :**

Oral : 15 mg capsules.

Dose : Adults : 15-30 mg at bed time.

Elderly : 15 mg at bed time.

Use : Hypnotic.

5. **Nitrazepam (Nitravet, Nitrosun) :**

Oral : 5, 10 mg tablets.

2.5 mg kid tablets.

Dose : Infants and children 2.5-5 mg at bed time

Adults 5-10 mg at bed time

Elderly 2.5-5 mg at bed time.

Use : Hypnotic.

Barbiturate

1. **Phenobarbitone (Gardenal, Luminal) :**

Oral : 30, 60 mg tablets.

Dose : Adults 30 mg at bed time.

Use : Hypnotic, Anticonvulsant.

Cyclopyrrolone derivative

1. **Zopiclone (Zopicone) :**

Oral : 7.5 mg film coated tablets.

Dose : Adults : 7.5-15 mg at bed time.

Elderly : 3.75 mg at bed time.

Use : Hypnotic.

Pharmacists should advise the patients regarding the following properties of sedative-hypnotics

1. Drinking alcoholic beverages enhance the effect of sedative hypnotics.

2. Drowsiness may persist the next day after the use of barbiturate or zopiclone, therefore they should avoid driving or operating heavy machines.

Contraindications

Barbiturates and benzodiazepines are contraindicated in porphyria.

EXPERIMENT NO. 20

Effect of chlorpromazine in rats

AIM

To study the property of chlorpromazine to block conditioned avoidance response.

PRINCIPLE

Dopamine is one of the neurotransmitters present in the central nervous system. Excessive dopaminergic activity produces symptoms of psychosis. Drugs which increase dopaminergic activity aggravate psychosis (e.g. l-dopa acts as a precursor of dopamine, amphetamine acts as a releaser of dopamine and apomorphine acts as a D_2-receptor agonist). Because of the dopamine agonist activity apomorphine induces stereotype behaviour in animal. Antipsychotics (Neuroleptics) inhibit apomorphine induced stereotype behaviour. Inhibition or blockade of Conditioned Avoidance Response (CAR) is one of the most reliable tests of antipsychotic action. Chlorpromazine exhibits antipsychotic effect by acting as a Dopamine D_2-receptor antagonist.

EQUIPMENTS AND OTHER MATERIALS REQUIRED

Cooks pole climbing apparatus, rat cages, disposable needles and syringes.

Description about Cook's pole-climbing response apparatus

It has an experimental chamber with floor-grid in a sound proofed enclosure. The enclosure has a clear perspex sliding door. Inbuilt arrangement for both types of stimuli, buzzer and shock which may be presented singly or together just by pressing a button for an internally timed duration of 30 seconds, which may be terminated any time by pressing another button. The duration of the stimuli may also be manually controlled for any desired period.

The pole is in two portions and should be screwed in the small lid on the top of the apparatus so that the smaller portion (handle) is outside the lid. The pole can be withdrawn along with the lid to remove the animal. Raising the front door upwards will allow an animal to be introduced into or removed from the chamber.

Animal

Albino rat.

Drug solutions required

1. Normal saline.
2. Chlorpromazine hydrochloride 2 mg/mL.

PROCEDURE

1. Select 12 albino rats having body weight between 80-120 g (male rat or non-pregnant female rats).
2. Keep one rat at a time in the chamber of Cook's pole climbing apparatus.
3. Give a series of foot shocks (80 volts - 5 pulse/sec) and buzzer for 30 seconds.
4. Observe whether the rat manages to climb the pole, where it does not get the shock.
5. Repeat the delivery of shock and buzzer for 30 seconds at 2 hours interval and train each rat 3 times a day.
6. Give the training for a week for all 12 rats.
7. After a week training expose each rat to buzzer only. If the rat climbs the pole within 30 seconds it indicates that Conditioned Avoidance Response (CAR) is established.
8. If any rat does not respond to buzzer continue the training till the CAR is established.
9. Divide the rats into 2 groups of six animals.
10. Weigh the rat in each group do the marking and keep them in rat cages.
11. Place each rat in the chamber of Cook's pole climbing apparatus.
12. Deliver the buzzer stimuli and observe the time taken by each rat in both groups for climbing the pole.
13. Administer the drug solutions as given below :

    Group I : Normal saline 1 mL/kg i.p.

    Group II : Chlorpromazine hydrochloride 2 mg/kg i.p.
14. After 30 minutes record the observation as shown below.

Group I : Control Normal Saline 1 mL/kg i.p.

S. No.	Markings	Body weight	Dose in ml	Time of injection	Observations Time required for climbing the pole Before drug	After drug
1.	Head	120	0.12	10 am	3 sec	3 sec
2.	Back	110	0.11	-	2 sec	2 sec
3.	Tail	100	0.1	-	3 sec	3 sec
4.	F limb	120	0.12	-	2 sec	2 sec
5.	H. limb	120	0.12	-	3 sec	3 sec
6.	Head & back	100	0.1	-	2 sec	2 sec

Group II : Chlorpromazine hydrochloride 2 mg/kg i.p. (2 mg/ mL)

S. No.	Markings	Body weight	Dose in ml	Time of injection	Observations Time required for climbing the pole Before drug	After drug
1.	Head	110	0.11	11 am	3 sec	None of the
2.	Back	120	0.12	-	2 sec	animals climbed
3.	Tail	100	0.1	-	3 sec	the pole when
4.	F. limb	120	0.12	-	3 sec	buzzer was on
5.	H. limb	100	0.1	-	2 sec	
6.	Head & back	120	0.12	-	3 sec	

OBSERVATION AND CONCLUSION

1. Chlorpromazine blocked the CAR (Conditioned Avoidance Response).
2. Chlorpromazine produced taming effect in rats.
3. Drugs which are likely to produce antipsychotic effect can be screened by this method.

Things to remember

Chlorpromazine is an antipsychotic agent. Drugs available for the treatment of psychosis are as follows :

1. **Chlorpromazine hydrochloride :**

   Oral : 10, 25, 50, 100, 200 mg tablets.

Parenteral : 250 mg/mL.

Dose : 25-800 mg/day in severe psychosis.

2. **Fluphenazine decanoate (Anatensol) :**
   Parenteral : 25 mg/mL.
   Dose : 25 mg i.m. every 2-4 weeks.

3. **Haloperidol (Depidol, Halidol, Halopidol) :**
   Oral : 5, 10, 20 mg tablets.
   Dose : 5-20 mg/day.
   Parenteral : Haloperidol decanoate 50 mg/mL.
   Dose : 1 ml in every 15-30 days.
   Haloperidol 5 mg tab + Benzhexol 2 mg tab
   Haloperidol 5 mg tab + Trihexyphenidyl hydrochloride 2 mg tab
   Dose : 1 tab three times in a day/as required.

4. **Flupenthixol dihydrochloride (Fluanxol) :**
   Oral : 0.5, 1 and 3 mg tablets.
   Dose : Adult : 0.5-3 mg/day.
   Flupenthixol decanoate (Fluanxol depot)
   Parenteral : 20 mg/mL; 40 mg/mL
   Adult *Dose* : 20-40 mg/day
   Elderly patient : ½ to 1/4th of Adult dose.

5. **Loxapine succinate (Loxapac) :**
   Oral : 10 mg, 25 mg capsules.
   Adult *Dose* : 10 mg twice in a day.
   Loxapine hydrochloride
   Oral : 25 mg/ml.

6. **Pimozide (Larap) (Neurap) (Orap) :**
   Oral : 4 mg tablets.
   Dose : 2-12 mg/day.
   Contraindicated in arrhythmias.

7. **Thioridazine hydrochloride (Tensaril) (Thioril) :**
   Oral : 10, 25, 50, 100 mg tablets.
   Dose : Adult : Neurotics : 10-20 mg/day.
   Psychotics : 100-600 mg/day.
   Children : 0.5-2 mg/kg/day.

8. **Trifluoperazine hydrochloride (Trazine-S) :**
   Oral : 5 mg tab.
   Dose : 5 mg three times daily.

9. **Trifluperidol hydrochloride (Triperidol) :**
   Oral : 0.5 mg tablets.
   Dose : 0.5 mg/day.
   Parenteral : 2.5 mg/ml injection.
   Dose : 0.5-2.5 mg i.m. injection.

EXPERIMENT NO. 21

Hypnosis potentiating effect of chlorpromazine in mice

AIM

To study the influence of chlorpromazine on the pentobarbitone induced sleeping time in mice.

PRINCIPLE

Pentobarbitone is a barbiturate which increases the duration of opening of the chloride channel. It also inhibits the excitatory AMPA (DL alpha amino 3-hydroxy 5-methylisoxazole 4 propionate) glutamate receptors. Therefore, pentobarbitone acts as a central nervous system depressant.

Chlorpromazine is a neuroleptic which blocks dopamine D_2 receptors and produces calmness of the mental activity. Therefore, chlorpromazine potentiates the pentobarbitone induced sleeping time.

EQUIPMENTS AND OTHER MATERIALS REQUIRED

Stop watch, mouse cages, disposable needles and disposable syringes.

Animal   Albino mice.

Drug solutions required

Normal saline (Sodium Chloride 0.9 w/v).

Pentobarbitone sodium 4 mg/mL.

Chlorpromazine 0.3 mg/mL.

PROCEDURE

1. Select 20 albino mice having body weight between 25-30 g.
2. Fast the mice for 12 hours before the experiment.
3. Divide the mice into four groups of five animals.
4. Weigh the mouse in each group, do the marking and keep them in plastic cages.
5. Administer the drug solutions as shown below.

Group I : Normal saline 1 ml/100 g i.p.

Group II : Pentobarbitonesodium 45 mg/kg i.p. (Prepare 4.5 mg/ mL solution and inject 1 mL/100 g body weight).

Group III : Chlorpromazine 3 mg/kg i.p. (Prepare 0.3 mg/mL solution of chlorpromazine and inject 1 mL/100 g body weight).

Group IV : Administer chlorpromazine 3 mg/kg i.p. After 30 minutes administer pentobarbitone 45 mg/kg i.p.

6. Record the observations as shown below :

Group I : Normal saline 1 ml/kg i.p.

S. No.	Markings	Body weight	Dose	Time of injection	Motor activity	Sedation	LRR
					Observations		
1.	Head	25					
2.	Back	30					
3.	Tail	30					
4.	Head & back	30					
5.	Head & tail	30					

LRR = Loss of Righting Reflexd.

Make similar tables for Group II, Group III and Group IV.

OBSERVATIONS AND CONCLUSIONS

1. Behaviour and motor activity of mice were normal in the group which received saline.

2. There was loss of righting reflex of the mice in the group which received pentobarbitone sodium. The duration of sleep was 30 minutes.

3. The spontaneous motor activity of the mice was reduced in the group which received chlorpromazine.

4. The group which received chlorpromazine and pentobarbitone sodium the duration of sleep was more than 30 minutes.

5. The above observations indicate that chlorpromazine potentiates the effects of pentobarbitone.

Things to remember

Antipsychotic agents enhance the sedative and hypnotic effect of barbiturates. Alcohol also enhances the sedative effect of barbiturates. Patients should be advised not to take these drugs together.

CHAPTER 9
Antihistaminics

EXPERIMENT NO. 22

Effect of diphenhydramine in experimentally produced asthma in guinea pigs

AIM

To demonstrate the antagonistic effects of diphenhydramine against histamine—induced bronchospasm in the guinea-pig.

PRINCIPLE

Asthma is characterized by bronchospasm and difficulty in breathing. The above effects are mediated by autocoids like histamine, leukotrienes platelet activating factor, serotonin, kinins, etc. Guinea pig is very sensitive to histamine. When guinea pig is exposed to histamine vapour it exhibits bronchospasm, difficulty in breathing and convulsion. These effects of histamine are mediated through the action of histamine on H_1 receptors. Diphenhydramine is a H_1-receptor blocker. Therefore, diphenhydramine prevents the bronchospasm induced by histamine.

EQUIPMENTS AND OTHER MATERIALS REQUIRED

Histometer, stop watch, disposable needle and syringes.

Animal : Guinea pigs.

Drug solutions required

1. Normal saline.
2. Diphenhydramine 5 mg/mL.
3. Histamine diphosphate 30 µg/ml.

PROCEDURE

1. Select 4 guinea pigs having body weight between 250-350 g.
2. Fast the guinea pigs for 12 hours before the experiment.
3. Divide the guinea pigs into 2 groups of 2 animals each.
4. Weigh the guinea pigs in each group and mark them for identification.

5. Administer the drug solutions as shown below.

   Group I : Normal saline 1 ml/kg i.p.

   Group II : Diphenhydramine 5 mg/kg s.c.

6. One hour later place each guinea pig in histamine chamber and replace the cover.

7. With the help of compressor, spray a finely atomized mist of histamine diphosphate (30 µg/ml.) from neubulizer in both compartments (compressor pressure 100 mmHg to operate neubulizer).

8. Using a stop watch record the time of histamine administration.

9. Observe the signs of respiratory distress (difficulty and cessation of breathing, asphyxial convulsion) and the animal falling on its side.

10. Record the observations as shown below.

   Group I : Normal saline 1 ml/kg.

S. No.	Marking	Weight of G. pig	Dose	Time of administration histamine	Time of appearance of respiratory distress	Remarks
1.	Head	250	0.25			
2.	Back	300	0.3			

Make similar table for Group II also.

OBSERVATIONS AND CONCLUSIONS

1. The normal saline treated group showed respiratory distress (Bronchospasm) within 2 minutes period.

2. The guinea pigs in the group II which are treated with diphenhydramine did not show respiratory distress for more than 10 minutes.

3. The above observations indicate that diphenhydramine antagonises the actions and effects of histamine.

Things to remember

1. Diphenhydramine is a H_1-receptor blocker used in allergic reactions. Other H_1-blockers are also used in allergic reactions.

PATHOPHYSIOLOGY OF ASTHMA

Asthma is an immunological disorder mediated by reaginic IgE antibodies. IgE antibodies are bound to mast cells present in the lungs (airway mucosa). Whenever an antigen combines with IgE antibodies, release of autocoids like histamine, leukotrienes, platelet activating factor (PAF), prostaglandins, thromboxanes etc. occurs. These autocoids cause bronchoconstriction. Therefore, either the drugs which prevent the release of autocoids or the drug which prevent the actions of autocoids are used in the treatment of asthma in clinical practice. The following drugs are widely used in the treatment of asthma.

Beta-2 receptor agonists

1. **Albuterol (Salbutamol, Asthalin, Salbetol) :**
   Oral : 2, 4, 8 mg tablets; 2 mg/5 ml syrup.
   Dose : Child under 2 years : 100 micrograms/kg 4 times daily.
   2-6 years : 1-2 mg 3-4 times daily.
   6-12 years : 2 mg 3-4 times daily.
   Parenteral : 50, 500, 1000 micrograms/mL.
   Aerosolinhalation : Child 100 micrograms (1 puff).
   Adult 200 micrograms (2 puffs).
   Inhalation of powder : Child 200 micrograms.
   Adult 200-400 micrograms.

2. **Salmeterol xinafoate (Salmeter) :**
   Inhalation : 25 micrograms/Inhalation.
   Dose : Children below 4 years not recommended.
   Children over 4 years 50 micrograms twice in a day.
   Adults : 100 micrograms (4 puffs) twice in a day.

3. **Terbutaline sulphate (Bricanyl) :**
   Oral : 5 mg tablets, 2.5 mg tablets; 1.5 mg/mL syrup.
   Dose : Children under 3 years 750 micrograms 3 times in a day.
   3-7 years 0.75-15 mg 3 times in a day.
   7-15 years 1.5-3 mg 3 times in a day.
   Inhalation : 250 microgram per metered dose inhaler 1-2 inhalations 3-4 times daily.
   Injection : 0.5 mg per ml.

Child : 2-15 years 10 micrograms/kg by subcutaneous, intramuscular or slow intravenous injection. Slow intravenous infusion 3-5 micrograms/mL.

Adult : 0.5 mg s.c. 4 times in a day.

Antimuscarinic bronchodilators

Ipratropium bromide (Ipravent) :

Inhalation : 20 micrograms/metered inhalation.

Dose : Children 3-6 years 1 puff (20 micrograms) 3 times in a day.

Adults : 1-2 puffs (20 micrograms/puff) 3-4 times in a day.

Mast cell stabilizers

Sodium cromoglycate (Cromal-5 inhaler, Fintal inhaler, Ifiral):

Inhaler : 1, 5 mg per metered dose inhaler. Two inhalations 4 times in a day.

Cartridge : 20 mg.

Dose : Initial 4 caps inhaled per day 4 times in a day. Maintenance 1 cap/day.

Nedocromil sodium :

Inhalation : 2 mg per metered inhalation.

Dose : 4 mg (2 puffs) twice daily.

Corticosteroids

Beclomethasone dipropionate (Becoride) :

Inhalation : 50, 100, 250 micrograms per activation.

Dose : Children over 4 years of age upto 400 micrograms per day in divided doses.

Adults and children over 12 years :

Mild asthma 200-500 micrograms/day.

Moderate asthma 600-1000 micrograms/day.

Severe asthma 1000-2000 micrograms/day.

Dexamethasone phosphate (Decicort) :

Tablets : 500 micrograms.

Injection : 4 mg/2 mL.

Oral : Adults 500 micrograms/day.

Dose by oral/injection should be adjusted according to the clinical conditions.

Budesonide (Bude cort inhaler, Budecort respules) :

Inhalation : 50, 100, 200, 250, 500 micrograms per metered dose inhaler.

Dose : Children 0.25 mg-0.5 mg twice in a day.

Adults : 0.5-1 mg twice in a day. Maximum 1-2 mg twice in a day.

Xanthine derivative

Theophylline (anhydrons) (Broncordil, Theolong) :

Oral : 100, 200, 300 mg tablets.

80 mg/15 mL Elixir.

100 mg/5 mL syrup.

Dose : Children 1-9 years 16-24 mg/kg/day.

Adults : 400 mg in 2 divided doses. Maximum dose 13 mg/kg ₁ body weight.

Etophylline 77 mg + Theophylline 23 mg (Deriphyllin) :

Tablets.

Dose : 1-3 tablets thrice in a day.

Deriphylline sustained release preparations (Tablets) :

Deriphylline 150 mg (contains Etophylline 115 mg + Theophylline 35 mg).

Deriphylline 300 mg (combines Etophylline 231 mg + Theophylline 69 mg).

Deriphylline 450 mg (contains Etophylline 346 mg + Theophylline 104 mg).

Dose : 1 tab twice in a day.

Deriphylline syrup :

Paediatric : Etophylline 46.5 mg + Theophylline 14 mg/5 mL syrup.

Dose : 1-9 years : 16-24 mg/kg/day individed doses.

CHAPTER 10
PyrogenTesting

EXPERIMENT NO. 23

Evaluation technique to identify the presence of pyrogens in parenteral preparations

AIMS

A. To detect the presence of bacterial endotoxins (pyrogens) in parenterals using rabbit.

PRINCIPLE

Rabbits are very sensitive to pyrogens. Therefore, when pyrogen containing solution is given intravenously it produces a rise in body temperature within 3 hours. If the parenteral solution is sterile it does not produce any rise in temperature. If the sample produces a rise in temperature (2.4° C) from the mean value then the sample is considered pyrogenic and discarded.

APPARATUS REQUIRED

Rabbit cages, Telethermometer (sensitivity ± 0.1° C), Disposable needle and syringes.

Animal required

Healthy rabbits having body weight not less than 1.5 kg.

PROCEDURE

1. Select healthy rabbits and keep them in the animal room maintained at a temperature of 22 ± 2° C for 3 weeks period.

2. Feed the rabbits with pellet diet and filtered drinking water.

3. Perform 'Sham test' in an airconditioned room (i.e. inject pyrogen free isotonic solution (10 ml/kg, i.v.) and record the rectal temperature using telethermometer for 3 hours at 30 minutes interval.

4. Give 3 days rest for all rabbits.

5. Record the initial temperature for each rabbit at 30 minutes interval for a period of 90 minutes. Do not select rabbits having initial temperature above 39.8° C and below 38° C.

6. Administer the preparation to be tested for pyrogen by intravenous route (10 mL/kg) through the marginal ear vein.

7. Record the temperature for each rabbit at 30 minutes intervals for a period of 3 hours.

8. Find out the difference between initial temperature and final temperature for each rabbit. This is taken to be its response.

9. Interpret the results as given below :

Number of rabbits	Material passes if summed response does not exceed	Material fails if the summed response exceeds
3	1.15	2.65
6	2.8	4.3
9	4.45	5.95
12	6.60	6.60

Significances of rabbit pyrogen test

Rabbit pyrogen test is conducted for products such as :

Antitoxins

Antivenins

Blood derivatives

Immune serums

Immunologic diagnostic aids

Toxoids

Vaccines

B. To detect bacterial endotoxins in human drugs, parenterals; Veterinary drugs and medical devices using Limulus Amebocyte Lysate test (LAL Test)

PRINCIPLE

In the year 1956 F.B. Bang observed that the Limulus Amebocyte Lysate which is obtained from aqueous extracts of the circulating amebocytes of the horse shoe crab (*Limulus polyphemus*) has the unique property of reacting with Endotoxin and forms a firm clot. Young, Levin and Pendergast later demonstrated such reaction to be enzymatic.

The Limulus Amebocyte Lysate is prepared from the blood of *Limulus polyphemus* (Horse shoe crab) without killing the crab. The Limulus Amebocyte Lysate is mixed with the test sample and incubated at 37° C for 1 hour. Appearance of clear visible clot indicates the presence of Endotoxin. If it remains fluid it indicates the absence of Endotoxin.

The determination of the reaction end point is made with dilution from material under test in direct comparison with parallel dilutions of a reference endotoxin and the quantities of endotoxin are expressed in defined endotoxins units.

Sensitivity of LAL test

LAL test detects 0.1‹ ng of Endotoxin/mL.

Apparatus required

Incubator, Autoclave, Glasspipet 0.1 ml, Serological 0.5 mL, Dry oven, Test tube rack, needles, Micropipet, Stop watch, pH meter, 10 x 75 mm pyrogen free tube.

Reagents required

1. Limulus amebocyte lysate (orlysate) : Lysed preparation from circulating amebocyte of the crabs buffered, packed lyophilized and sealed. This is to be reconstituted with pyrogen free distilled water.

   Storage condition for orlysate : Store at 5° C. Protect from light (sunlight). Reconstituted orlysate should be used within 48 hours. Store in deep freezer (- 30 to - 40° C).

2. Pyrogen free water.

3. Control Standard Endotoxin (CSE).

PROCEDURE

A. Preparation

Keep the LAL test room sterile. Sterilise the glass materials by autoclaving at 20 PSI for 3 hours followed by dry heating at 180° C for 4 hours. Samples should be collected at various stages of production according to requirement.

B. Preparing sample

1. Adjust the pH of the sample material between pH 6-8 with pyrogen free hydrochloric acid or sodium hydroxide of 0.1 M at room temperature.

2. Take 200 microliter of sample in a pyrogen free (75 x 10 mm) glass tube.

   Add 200 microliter of Limulus Amebocyte Lysate (orlysate) and mix gently. Incubate for 60 minutes at 37° C. A firm gel will indicate the presence of pyrogen in the product.

C. Positive control

Take 200 microliter of Limulus Amebocyte Lysate (orlysate) in a 75 x 10 mm glass test tube. Add 200 microliter of 0.5 xu of standard endotoxin. Mix gently and incubate at 37° C for 60 minutes. Observe the formation of Firm Gel.

Note : If gel does not appears after 1 hour it indicates that the Lysate is denatured.

D. Negative control

Take 200 microliter of pyrogen free water in a pyrogen free 75 x 10 mm tube. Add 200 microliter of Limulus Amebocyte Lysate (orlysate). Mix gently and incubate at 37°C for 60 minutes. Observe the tube for gel formation (A firm gel will not form, because there is no endotoxin).

Interpretation of test

After incubation for 1 hour, remove tubes from the incubator and gently invert at 180°. Appearance of a firm gel sticking inside indicates a clear positive test. A positive test indicates the presence of pyrogen. If the product gives a positive test, repeat the test 10 times.

A negative test means the product is free from pyrogens (anything less than a firm gel should be interpreted as negative e.g. soft weak gel, cloudy fluid heavy floculate).

USP recommended test

Take 12 tubes (75 x 10 mm) and arrange as given below :

A. 2 tubes for same product.

B. 2 tubes for negative control.

C. 2 tubes for positive control.

D. 6 tubes for EDS (Endotoxin dilution series).

Endotoxin dilution series

Take 6 tubes (75 x 10 mm) and add reagents as given below :

In tube No. 1 : Take 0.2 ml of LAL (orlysate). Add 0.2 ml of Endotoxin of 0.5 IU/ml.

In tube No. 2 : Take 0.2 ml of LAL (orlysate). Add 0.2 ml of Endotoxin of 0.25 IU/ml.

In tube No. 3 : Take 0.2 ml of LAL (orlysate). Add 0.2 ml of Endotoxin of 0.125 IU/ml.

In tube No. 4 : Take 0.2 ml of LAL (orlysate). Add 0.2 ml of Endotoxin 0.062 IU/ml.

In tube No. 5 : Take 0.2 ml of LAL (orlysate). Add 0.2 ml of Endotoxin 0.031 IU/ml.

In tube No. 6 : Take 0.2 ml of LAL (orlysate). Add 0.2 ml of Endotoxin 0.015 IU/ml.

Test for surgical devices

Surgical devices and attachments be washed/dipped in pyrogen free water in a pyrogen free container. The rinsing scheme as mentioned in USP is followed to avoid greater dilution of endotoxin.

Comparison between Rabbit pyrogen test Vs. LAL test

Rabbit pyrogen test	*LAL test*
1. Animal house required	Animal house not required
2. Biological	Chemical
3. Debatable	Clear, visible to naked eye
4. Expensive	Less expensive
5. In vivo	In vitro
6. Requires long preparation	Very short
7. Quantification not possible	Possible
8. Subjective test	Objective test
9. Time required for test 4 hours	Time required for test 1 hour
10. Ideal for vaccines, toxoids, antivenins etc.	Ideal for preparations other than vaccines, toxoids etc.

Applications of LAL test

1. *In the pharmaceutical industry* LAL test can be used to detect the presence of pyrogens in the parenteral preparations.

2. *Clinical applications* :

   (i) LAL test can be used to identify contaminated fluid or fluid injecting devices and attachments.

   (ii) Diagnosis of gram negative meningitis, arthritis.

   (iii) LAL test can be used to identify toxins present in food products, infant food and drinking water.

Caution

1. LAL sensitivity is enhanced by certain products and may give false positive test. In such cases conduct Rabbit pyrogen test.

2. Use siliconised glassware or polysterene containers because glass absorbs endotoxins and may give erratic result.

3. Do not use brown coloured (denatured) lysate.

CHAPTER 11

Absorption of Drugs

EXPERIMENT NO. 24

Study of drug absorption in vitro (Transport of drug across the cell membrane)

AIM

To study the transport of glucose (or other drugs) across the intestinal membrane of the isolated guinea pig ileum.

PRINCIPLE

Absorption is a process by which a drug enters body fluids. Absorption of drugs involves their passage across cell membranes. Biological membranes consist of lipids and proteins. They are highly selective permeability barrier. Membrane lipids are relatively small molecules. They have both hydrophilic and hydrophobic moiety. Proteins serve as pumps, gates, receptors, energy transducers and enzymes.

Drugs are transported across cell membrane by various mechanisms which are as follows :

1. **Passive transfer :**	2. **Specialized transport :**
(a) Simple diffusion	(a) Active transport
(b) Filtration	(b) Facilitated diffusion
	(c) Pinocytosis

Simple diffusion

Dissolution of a lipid-soluble molecules in the lipid portion of the cell membrane and thereafter diffusing across the barrier. Drugs move across the membrane from a region of higher concentration to an area of lower drug concentration until equilibrium is reached e.g. Ether, nitrous oxide.

Filtration

Cell membranes have channels or pores that allow small water soluble molecules and ions (sodium, potassium, chloride) to pass through by simple filtration.

e.g. Filtration of drugs through the glomerular membrane of the kidney.

Specialized transport

(a) Active transport

Active transport refers to transport of substances against a concentration or electrochemical gradient e.g. Penicillins are actively secreted into the urine.

(b) Facilitated diffusion

It is a special form of carrier transport that has many characteristics of active transport, except that the substrate does not move against a concentration gradient e.g. uptake of glucose by cells.

Pinocytosis

It refers to the ability of cells to engulf small droplets e.g. gentamicin enters the proximal tubule of the kidney by this mechanism.

EQUIPMENTS AND OTHER ITEMS REQUIRED

Thermostatic student organ bath, oxygen cylinder, surgical instruments, spectrocolorimeter, glucose kits, micropipette.

Animal required

Guinea pig.

Physiological solution

Ringer solution.

PROCEDURE

1. Anaesthetize the guinea pig using suitable inhalation anaesthetic like ether.
2. Cut open the abdomen and expose the intestine region.
3. Cut off two pieces of ileum portion (10 cm length) and keep them in Ringer's solution at 37°C and clean with Ringer solution using tuberculin syringe.
4. Tie one end of the open intestine with silk thread.

5. Remove the Ringer solution from the lumen of the intestine.

6. Take a needle having a dull end (tip cut off) and introduce it to the other open end of the ileum and tie firmly with it as shown below :

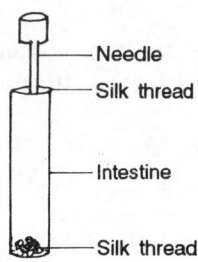

7. Fill the intestinal bag with Ringer solution containing 0.3% glucose using a syringe attached to the needle.

8. Mount the tissue in the inner organ bath containing Ringer's solution (Sodium chloride 9.5 g, Potassium chloride 0.2 g, Magnesium chloride 0.2 g, Sodium bicarbonate 0.2 g, distilled water upto 1000 ml) as shown below :

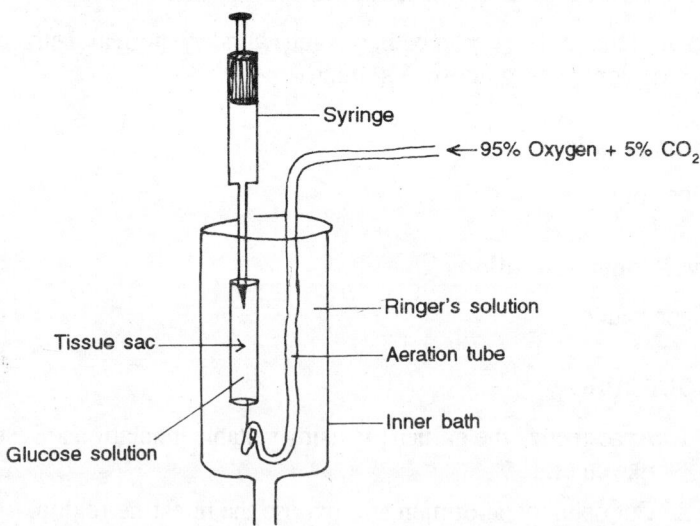

9. Oxygenate the Ringer solution with 95% oxygen and 5% carbondioxide.

10. Withdraw samples after 15, 30, 45, 60 and 90 minutes from the inner organ bath fluid surrounding the ileum. Also take the sample from the ileum bag at 90 minute.

11. Analyse the glucose concentrations in the samples.

Procedure for everted sac

1. Take the 2nd piece of ileum in a petri dish containing Ringer's solution.

2. Insert a glass rod having diameter equal to the diameter of the lumen of the ileum and evert it to get the mucosa (inside) to the outside.

3. Then follow the steps 4 to 11 as described for the normal ileum.

Calculate the ratios of glucose concentration between serosa and mucosa side and also mucosa and serosa side.

Plot the ratios of concentration of serosa/concentration of mucosa and concentration of mucosa/concentration of serosa versus time as shown below.

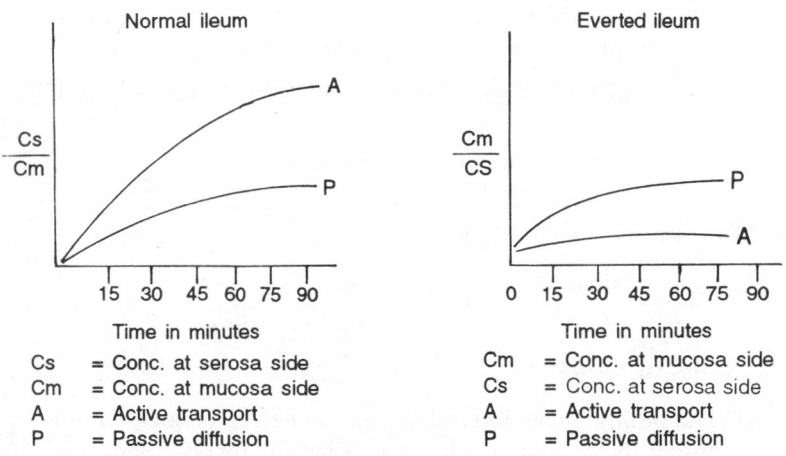

Normal ileum	Everted ileum
Cs = Conc. at serosa side	Cm = Conc. at mucosa side
Cm = Conc. at mucosa side	Cs = Conc. at serosa side
A = Active transport	A = Active transport
P = Passive diffusion	P = Passive diffusion

OBSERVATION AND CONCLUSION

Two mechanisms are responsible for the absorption of glucose :

(a) Active transport against a concentration gradient (A)

(b) Simple diffusion (P).

Therefore, in the normal guinea pig ileum the active transport process is prominent and when the ileum is everted there is little active transport. However, simple diffusion occurs in both cases.

CHAPTER 12

Bioassay

EXPERIMENT NO. 25

Bioassay is defined as the estimation of the nature, concentration or potency present in unit quantity of the test substance by measurement of the biological response that it produces.

Biological standardization is a process by which an unknown drug is compared and adjusted in terms of the standard.

Advantages and the uses of bioassays

1. One can measure the biological (the Pharmacological) activity of new or chemically undefined substances.
2. Substances which undergo decomposition during chemical assay can be estimated biologically without loss of potency.
3. To measure the therapeutic effectiveness of a new drug treatment.
4. To measure the toxicity of a new drug.

Disadvantages of bioassay

1. Biological variation
2. Time consuming
3. Costly
4. Cruelty to animals

Principles of bioassay

1. The biological activity of an unknown drug or chemical should always be compared with an internationally accepted standard.
2. The biological activity exhibited by the test compound in the living system should closely resemble the therapeutic activity of the drug, e.g. :
   (a) The bioassay of a cardiac glycoside should be done by measuring its activity on cardiac muscle, since cardiac glycoside is used in the congestive heart failure.
   (b) The bioassay of a new insulin preparation can be done by measuring the hypoglycemic effect of the new preparation in rabbits.

3. Species which show maximum sensitivity should be selected for the bioassay.

   For example : Guinea pig ileum is most sensitive to histamine.

4. The bioassay method should give reproducible results.

5. Bioassay should be designed properly in order to estimate error limits by statistical analysis.

Methods employed for bioassays

Two major types of bioassay are done in the laboratory :

1. Graded response bioassay

2. Quantal response bioassay.

Graded response bioassay (Quantitative dose effect relationship bioassay)

In graded response bioassay the dose of the drug is related to the size of the response produced in single biological unit. This graded response bioassay may be performed by the following methods :

(a) *Matching method* (comparative method, bracketting method, direct assay).

(b) *Indirect methods*.:

   (i) Graphical or interpolation method.

   (ii) Three point bioassay.

   (iii) Four point bioassay.

Direct bioassay (matching method) (comparative, bracketting method)

The aim of the matching method of bioassay is to determine the doses of the standard and unknown that produce the same response.

Example : Bioassay of acetylcholine by matching method using frog rectus abdominis muscle.

BIOASSAY OF ACETYLCHOLINE

(a) Bioassay of acetylcholine by comparative method using frog rectus abdominis muscle

AIM

To find out the potency (or concentration) of the test sample by comparing the doses of standard acetylcholine and test acetylcholine that produce the same response.

PRINCIPLE

Frog rectus abdominis muscle is a voluntary muscle. At the neuromuscular junction, a nerve impulse liberates acetylcholine from the nerve ending into the cleft between muscle and nerve fibre. This acetylcholine causes a depolarization of the muscle fibre which in turn sets of a muscle action potential and contration of muscle fibre. The muscle fibres of lower species like frog are multiply innervated, hence, nerve stimulation causes persistent depolarization and a prolonged slow contraction of the muscle. Local administration of acetylcholine also produces similar effect. Frog rectus abdominis muscle contains nicotinic (N_2) receptors. Acetylcholine acts as an agonist.

EQUIPMENTS AND OTHER MATERIALS REQUIRED

Student kymograph, student organbath, aeration tube, aerator, aeration tube holder, frontal writing lever, lever holder, screw clip, haemostatic forceps, mariottle bottle, rubber tubes, tuberculine syringes 26 No. needle, pithing needle, scissors, forceps, thread, plasticine, gram weight.

Animal required

Frog.

Physiological solution required

Frog Ringer solution.

DRUG SOLUTION REQUIRED

Acetylcholine standard solution 100 µg/ml.
Test solution of acetylcholine.

PROCEDURE

1. Set up the assembly for the above mentioned experiment.

2. Pith a frog by passing a pithing needle through the occipito-atlantic junction between the brain and the spinal cord. The stretching out of the limbs indicate that the pithing is proper.

3. Place the frog in a dissection tray.

4. Pick up the skin of abdomen with the help of forceps and make proper incision to expose the rectus abdominis muscle.

5. Cut along the margin of the rectus abdominis muscle and then make a transverse cut through the sternum just above the base.

6. Free the rectus abdominis muscle from the anterior abdominal vein.

7. Lift the muscle gently and divide the muscle longitudinally.

8. Tie a long thread on the upper side of the rectus muscle and a short thread on the lower side of the rectus abdominis muscle.

9. Transfer the muscle to a petridish containing frog Ringer solution.

10. Tie the short thread to the hook of the aeration tube and place the rectus muscle in the inner organ both containing frog Ringer solution.

11. Tie the long thread to a frontal writing lever. The load on the lever should be 1 gram. The magnification should be between 5-7 times.

12. Stabilize the rectus muscle for 55 minutes period.

13. During the stabilization period replace the frog Ringer solution in the inner organ bath at an interval of 5 minutes.

14. After stabilization for a period of 55 minutes switch on the kymograph and record the normal tracing for a period of 30 seconds. At the end of 30 seconds period inject 0.1 ml of acetylcholine solution into the inner organ bath and record the response for a period of 90 seconds (Drug contact time). At the end of 90 seconds switch off the kymograph and give 3-4 washings of rectus muscle with frog Ringer solution.

15. Inject 0.1 ml of acetylcholine solution into the inner organ bath once again and record the response for 90 seconds.

16. If two equipotent responses are observed with similar doses of acetylcholine, then record the response of acetylcholine with higher doses (0.2, 0.4, 0.8 and 1 ml) as shown below :

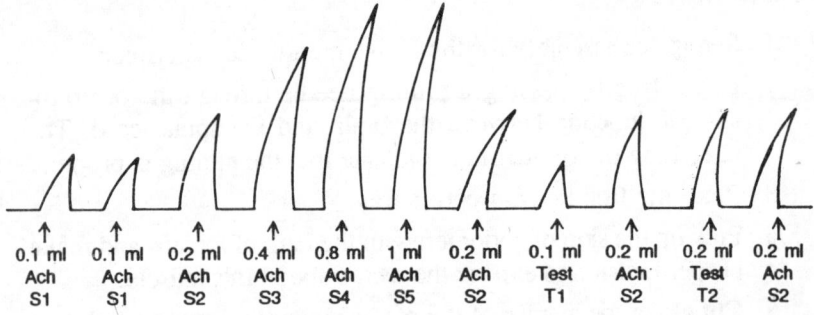

↑	↑	↑	↑	↑	↑	↑	↑	↑	↑	↑
0.1 ml	0.1 ml	0.2 ml	0.4 ml	0.8 ml	1 ml	0.2 ml	0.1 ml	0.2 ml	0.2 ml	0.2 ml
Ach	Ach	Ach	Ach	Ach	Ach	Ach	Test	Ach	Test	Ach
S1	S1	S2	S3	S4	S5	S2	T1	S2	T2	S2

17. Select a dose of the standard which produces submaximal response.

18. Administer the dose of the standard acetylcholine solution which produces submaximal response and record the response for 90 seconds.

19. Inject 0.1 ml of the test sample and record the response for 90 seconds and compare the response with that of the response produced by submaximal dose of the standard acetylcholine solution. Then administer either an increase dose or decrease dose of the test solution and record the responses till a response of the test matches with that of the submaximal response of the standard.

20. Find out the concentration of the test sample :

$$\text{Concentration of the test} = \frac{\text{Dose of the standard}}{\text{Dose of the test}} \times \text{Conc. of the standard}$$

Note : Students can perform the following experiments also in the laboratory.

1. Bioassay of acetylcholine by matching method using the following tissues namely : Leech muscle, Guinea pig ileum and rat intestine.

2. Bioassay of histamine by matching method using guinea pig ileum.

3. Bioassay of adrenaline by matching method using rabbit intestine.

4. Bioassay of oxytocin by matching method using rat uterus.

5. Bioassay of 5-hydroxytryptanine by matching method using rat fundus.

INDIRECT BIOASSAY

(b) Bioassay of acetylcholine by graphical method using frog rectus abdominis muscle

AIM

To find out the potency (or concentration) of the test sample by calculationg the matching doses of the standard and unknown indirectly from the graph.

REQUIREMENTS

Similar to part-a (Experiment No. 25)

PROCEDURE

1. Follow steps 1 to 16 of experiment No. 25 part a.

2. Inject 0.1 ml of the test sample and record the response for 90 seconds. If the smallest dose of the test sample produces a response which is similar to the response produced by the maximum dose of the standard acetylcholine then dilute the test sample for further administration.

3. Then administer a dose of the test sample which should produce a response more than that of the response produced by the smallest dose of standard acetylcholine and less than that of the response produced by the highest dose of standard acetylcholine.

4. Fix the graph and measure the height of contraction of the response produced by each dose of standard acetylcholine and test acetylcholine solution.

5. Plot a graph showing log dose of standard acetylcholine on X-axis and response on Y axis.

6. Measure the response (in mm) produced by the test sample and mark the point on Y axis. Then draw a horizontal line from the point on Y axis and then a perpendicular line from the point where the horizontal line meets the log dose-response curve as shown below.

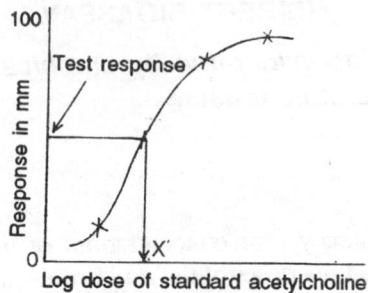

Log dose of standard acetylcholine

Find out the antilog of **X**.

For example if the antilog of x = 0.2 ml, and the test response is produced by 0.4 ml of the test solution, one can say that 0.2 ml of the standard is equal to 0.4 ml of the test.

Therefore, conc. of the test = $\dfrac{0.2}{0.4}$ × conc. of std.

Note : Graphical method of bioassay is preferred whenever volume of the test sample available is very less.

Note : Students can perform the following experiments also in the laboratory.

1. Bioassay of acetylcholine by graphical method using the following tissues namely : Leech muscle, guinea pig ileum and rat intestine.

2. Bioassay of histamine by graphical method using guinea pig ileum.

3. Bioassay of adrenaline by graphical method using rabbit intestine.

4. Bioassay of oxytoxin by graphical method using rat uterus.

5. Bioassay of 5-hydroxytryptamine by graphical method using rat fundus.

THREE-POINT BIOASSAY

(c) Bioassay of acetylcholine by 3 point bio-assay using frog rectus abdominis muscle

AIM

The aim of the three point bioassay is to find the dose of the test solution which produces the same response as that of a particular dose of the standard solution.

PROCEDURE

1. Set up the assembly for the frog rectus abdominis muscle preparation.

2. Record the dose-dependent effect of the standard solution of acetylcholine.

3. Select two doses of standard say s_1 and s_2 which produce submaximal response.

4. Select a dose of the test sample t_1 which is likely to produce a response less than the response produced by s_2 dose of the standard as shown below.

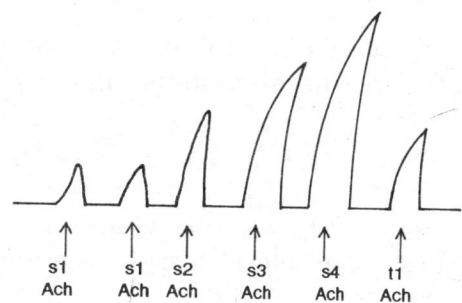

5. Measure the height of contraction produced by s_1 dose as S_1.

6. Measure the height of contraction produced by s_2 dose as S_2.

7. Measure the height of contraction produced by t_1 dose as T_1.

8. Calculate the potency of the test solution :

$$\text{Potency of test solution} = \frac{S_1}{t_1} \times \text{antilog} \left(\frac{T_1 - S_1}{S_2 - S_1} \times \log \frac{s_2}{s_2} \right)$$

A three point assay is occasionally useful when the test preparation is in very short supply.

Note : Students can perform the following experiments also in the laboratory.

1. Bioassay of acetylcholine by three-point bioassay method using the following tissues namely : Leech muscle, guinea pig ileum and rat intestine.

2. Bioassay of histamine by three-point bioassay method using guinea pig ileum.

3. Bioassay of oxytocin by three-point bioassay method using rat uterus.

4. Bioassay of adrenaline by three-point bioassay method using rabbit intestine.

5. Bioassay of 5-hydroxytryptamine by three-point bioassay method using rat fundus.

FOUR POINT BIOASSAY (PARALLEL LINE ASSAY)

In four point bioassay comparisons are based on analysis of dose-response curves and the matching doses of standard and unknown are calculated.

(d) Bioassay of acetylcholine by four-point bioassay method using frog rectus abdominis muscle preparation

AIM

To find out the potency ratio between the standard and test sample of acetylcholine solution by four point bioassay method using frog rectus abdominis muscle preparation.

REQUIREMENTS

Similar to experiment part (a). (Experiment No. 25).

PROCEDURE

1. Set up the assembly for the frog rectus abdominis muscle preparation.

2. Record the dose-dependent effect of the standard solution of acetylcholine as shown below :

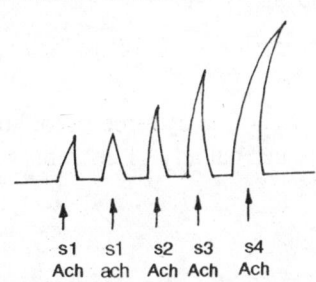

s1   s1   s2   s3   s4
Ach   ach   Ach Ach   Ach

3. Record the dose-dependent effect of the given test solution of acetylcholine as shown below :

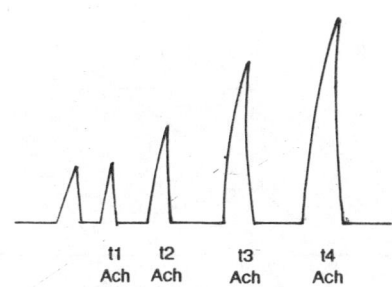

t1   t2   t3   t4
Ach   Ach   Ach   Ach

4. Select two doses of the standard solution of acetylcholine which produce submaximal responses (1 : 2 ratio preferably).

5. Select two doses of the test solution of acetylcholine which produce submaximal responses.

6. Administer the s_1, s_2, t_1 and t_2 doses four times in a randomised fashion (Latin square design).

s_1 = A; s_2 = B; t_1 = C; t_2 = D

1st sequence   ABCD

2nd sequence   BCDA

3rd sequence   CDAB

4th sequence   DABC

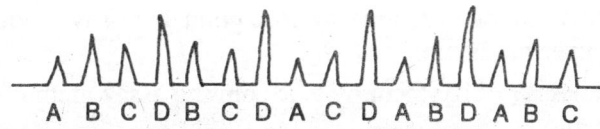

A   B   C   D   B   C   D   A   C   D   A   B   D   A   B   C

7. Measure the height of contraction produced by s_1(A) doses of acetylcholine and calculate the mean response as S1.

8. Measure the height of contraction produced by s_2 (B) doses of acetylcholine and calculate the mean response as S_2.

9. Measure the height of contraction produced t_1 (C) doses of acetylcholine and calculate mean response as T_1.

10. Measure the height of contraction produced by t_2 (D) doses of acetylcholine and calculate the mean response as T_2.

11. Plot a graph by taking log dose of the acetylcholine standard and test on x-axis and responses on y-axis as shown below :

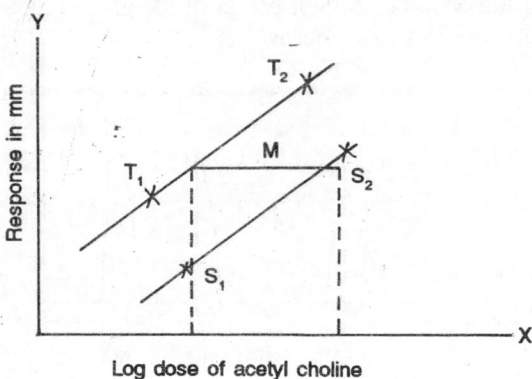

Log dose of acetyl choline

M = log potency ratio

Antilog of M = Potency ratio

12. Potency ratio can also be calculated using the formula :

$$\text{Potency ratio} = \frac{s_1}{t_1} \times \text{antilog} \left(\frac{T_2 - S_2 + T_1 - S_1}{T_2 - T_1 + S_2 - S_1} \times \log \frac{s_2}{s_1} \right)$$

Note : Students can perform the following experiments also in the laboratory.

1. Bioassay of acetylcholine by four-point bioassay method using the following tissues namely : Leech muscle, guinea pig ileum and intestine.

2. Bioassay of histamine by four-point bioassay method using guinea pig ileum.

3. Bioassay of oxytocin by four-point bioassay method using rat uterus.

4. Bioassay of 5-hydroxytryptamine by four-point-bioassay method using rat fundus.

Index